Laboratory Manual for Pharmacognosy

Dr. G. Sumalatha
M.Pharm, Ph.D

Associate Professor,

Department of Pharmacognosy

GBN Institute of Pharmacy

RangaReddy-501301, Telangana State

India

Copyright

All rights reserved. No part of this book may be reproduced or transmitted in any form or by any means, electronic or mechanical including photocopying, recording, or any information storage and retrieval system without the prior written permission from the publisher and the copyright holder.

Copyright © 2017-Dr. G.Sumalatha
All rights reserved.

ISBN-13: 978-1979555326
ISBN- 10:197955532X

CONTENTS

Pharmacognostic characters of some crude drugs

1. Belladonna
2. Cinchona
3. Physostigma
4. Nuxvomica
5. Senna
6. Rhubarb
7. Digitalis
8. Liquorice
9. Fenugreek
10. Linseed
11. Black mustard
12. Cinnamon
13. Clove
14. Ginger
15. Chamomile
16. Anise
17. Caraway
18. Fennel
19. Cardamom
20. Sage
21. Thyme
22. Peppermint oil
23. Capsicum

24. Vasaka
25. Rauwolfia
26. Datura
27. Carbohydrates

1. BELLADONNA LEAVES

Synonyms: Belladonnae folium, Deadly night shade leaf.
Latin name: *Atropa belladonna L.*
Family: *Solanaceae*

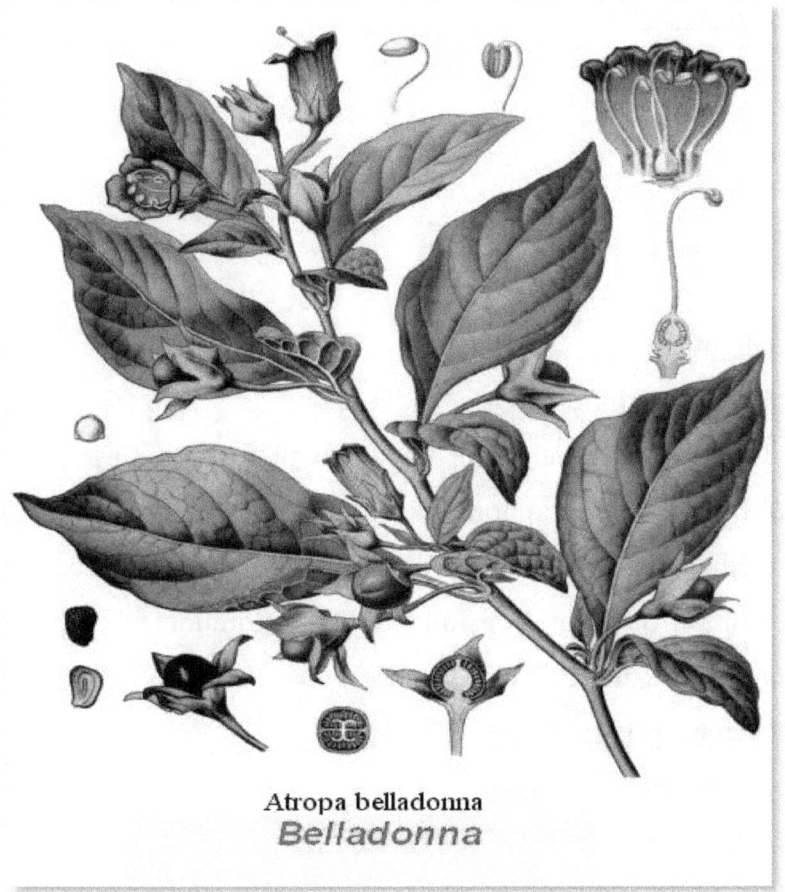

Atropa belladonna
Belladonna

- Perennial herbaceous plant (1m) height.
- Flowers pale purple.

1. Belladonna Leaves

- Fruits form berry and have black colour.
- The leaves are thin, long-pointed (acuminate).
- Odour: odorless.
- Taste: bitter.
- Origin: Central and Southern Europe.

Constituents

Alkaloids tropane group (0.4%)

1. Atropine
2. Hyoscyamine
3. Scopolamine
4. Hyoscine

Chemical test:

Vitali-Morin test:

The tropane alkaloid is treated with fuming nitric acid, followed by evaporation to dryness and addition of methanolic potassium hydroxide solution to an acetone solution of nitrated residue. Violet coloration takes place due to tropane derivative.

Pharmacological effects & Uses:

1. Atropine:

a) Antisecretory drug, so it used in: peptic ulcer therapy, gastritis, sinus nasal secretions, allergy and asthma.

b) Antispasmodic: decrease intestinal hyper motility.

1. Belladonna Leaves

c) Pupil dilator (mydriasis effect): used in the eyes surgery and in the

   eyes examinations.

d) Parasympatholytic agent, so it is used as antidote in case of poisoning from:

  1- Pilocarpine

  2- Physostigmine

  3- Organophosphate insecticides.

e) CNS stimulant (very dangerous to be used as CNS stimulant).

<u>2- Scopolamine</u> (CNS depressant): treatment of motion sickness (nausea &

   vomiting). antimuscarinic agent.

<u>3- Hyoscyamine</u>: control gastric secretions& intestinal hyper motility, so it is used

   in treatment of peptic ulcer and colic's.

<u>4- Hyoscine</u>: sedative effect used in case of colic's (renal and intestinal colic's).

Adulterants:

It is adulterated with *Phytolacca americana, Solanum nigrum and Ailanthus glandulosa.*

1. Belladonna Leaves

Microscopical examinations

Key elements:

1. Cuticular striation and numerous anisocytic stomata (2).
2. Glandular trichomes with uniseriate, multi-cellular stalks and unicellular heads (6).
3. Reticulate & thickened vessels (8).

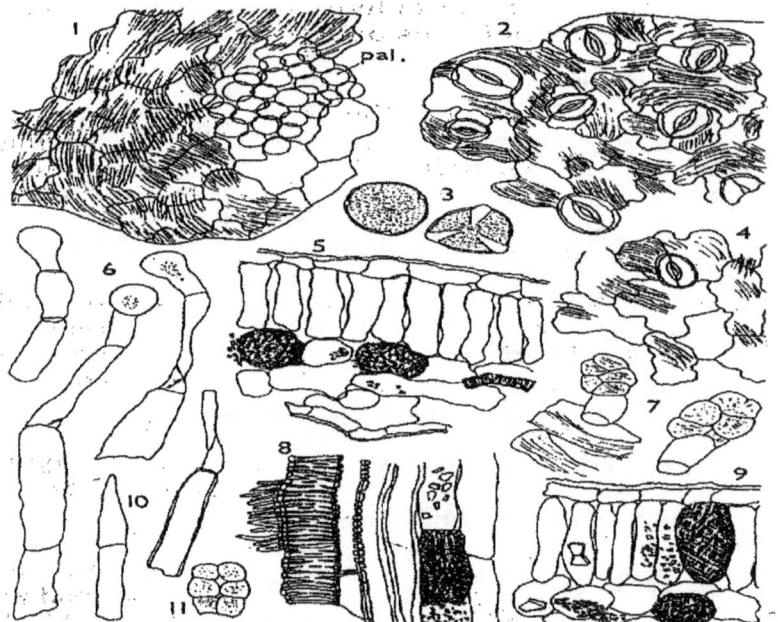

1. Upper epidermis in surface view showing cuticular striations and part of the underlying palisade (pal).
2. Lower epidermis in surface view showing cuticular striation and numerous anisocytic stomata.
3. Pollen grains.
4. Upper epidermis in surface view showing an anisocytic stoma.

1. Belladonna Leaves

5. Part of the lamina in sectional view, showing two idioblasts in the spongy mesophyll and scattered microsphenoidal crystals of calcium oxalate.
6. Glandular trichomes with uniseriate, multi-cellular stalks and unicellular heads.
7. Glandular trichomes with unicellular stalks and multicellular heads, one attached to a fragment of the epidermis over a vein.
8. Fragment of the inner tissues of the stem in longitudinal sectional view showing reticulately thickened vessels, xylem parenchyma, fibers and unlignified parenchymatous cells containing calcium oxalate crystals.
9. Part of the lamina in sectional view showing the upper epidermis, an idioblast in the palisade and other cells containing scattered prisms and microsphenoidal crystals of calcium oxalate.
10. Part of a covering trichome.
11. Multicellular head from a glandular trichome.

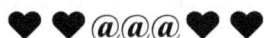

2. CINCHONA BARK:
CORTEX CINCHONAE:
CINCHONAE RUBRAE CORTEX

Synonyms: Jesuit's bark, Peruvian bark.
Latin name: *Cinchona succirubra. Pavon.* (Red Cinchona)
Family: *Rubiaceae*

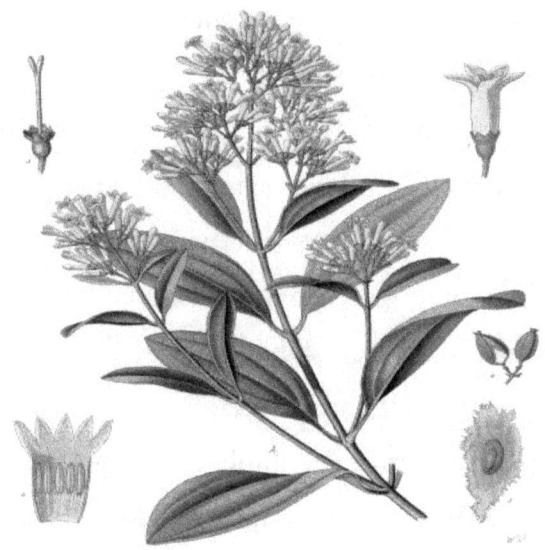

Cinchona succirubra

- ✓ Perennial trees 10m.
- ✓ The dried bark is curved ridges, greenish gray to brown.
- ✓ Origin: native to the tropical South America.

Constituent :

Alkaloids (quinine, quinidine, cinchonine).

2. Cinchona Bark

Chemical Tests :
1. Heat the powdered drug in a dried test tube with little glacial acetic acid, purple vapours are produced at the upper part of test tube.
2. **Thalleoquin test:** The powdered drug gives emerald green colour with bromine water and dilute ammonia solution.
3. Quinidine solution gives a white precipitate with silver nitrate solution, which is soluble in nitric acid.

Uses : Quinine: Antimalarial. Night muscles cramps.
Quinidine: Arrhythmias.

Substitutes:
Cuprea bark (*Remijia pedunculata*).

Microscopical examinations

Characteristic elements:
1. Cork (8).
2. Single fiber (1).
3. Cork and phelloderm in sectional view (5).
4. Parenchymatous cells containing starch granules and brown pigment (3).

2. Cinchona Bark

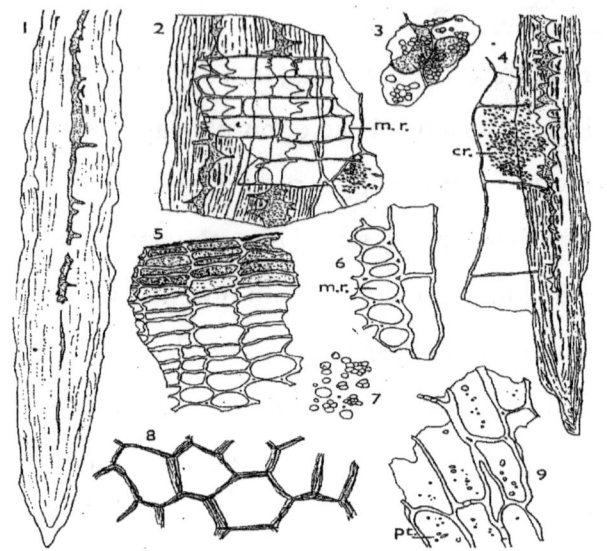

1. Part of a single fiber.
2. Part of a group of fibers and phloem parenchyma with overlying medullary ray (m.r.) in radial longitudinal section.
3. Parenchymatous cells containing starch granules and brown pigment.
4. Part of a fiber with phloem parenchyma, one cell containing calcium oxalate micro-crystals (Cr).
5. Cork and phelloderm in sectional view.
6. Phloem parenchyma and part of a medullary ray (m.r.) in tangential longitudinal section.
7. Starch granules.
8. Cork in surface view.
9. Phloem parenchyma with pits (pt.).

3. CALABAR BEAN: PHYSOSTIGMATIS SEMINA

Synonyms: Ordeal bean

Latin name: *Physostigma venenosum balfour.*

Family: *Leguminosae*

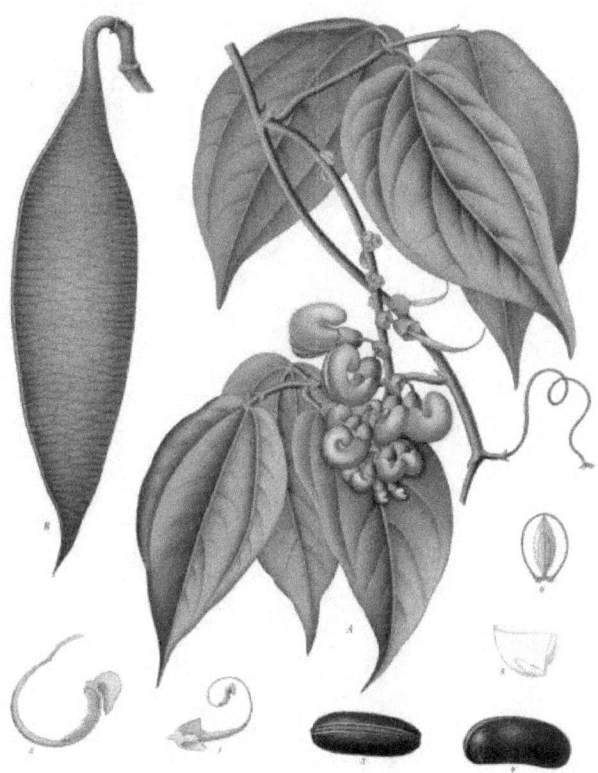

Calabar Bean

- ❖ Perennial climbing plant.
- ❖ Seeds: dark brown, oval, hard, odorless, bitter taste.

3. Calabar Bean

❖ Origin: West Africa, Calabar River.

Constituents:

Alkaloids- indole group:

1. Physostigmine (eserine) 0.04- 0.3%

2. Esreramine.

Uses:

- Increase intestinal motility and has myosis effect.
- Used to treat myasthenia gravis.

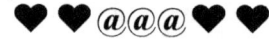

4. NUX VOMICA SEEDS: STRYCHNI SEMEN

Synonyms: Crow-fig

Latin name: *Strychnos nux-vomica Linne.*

Family: *Loganiaceae*

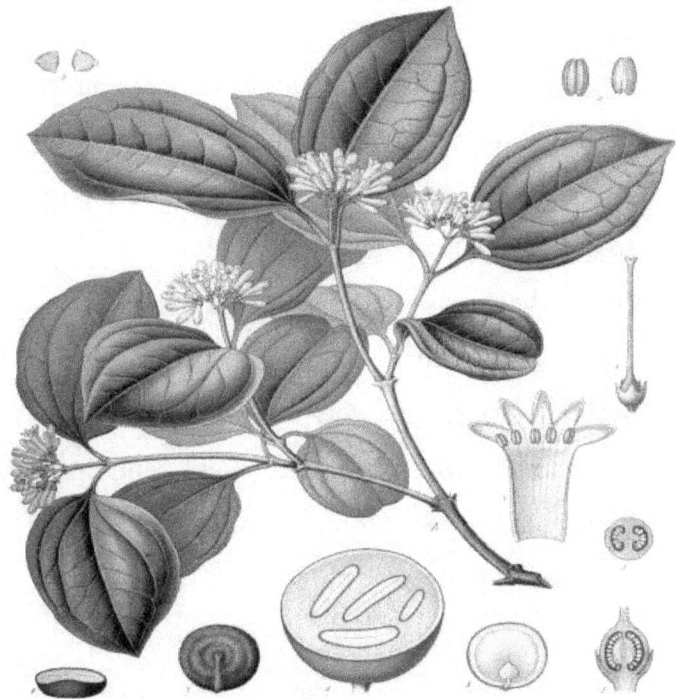

Strychnos nux-vomica

Nux-vomica: means a nut that causes vomiting.

- Perennial trees, 12m.
- Fruits form: berry 3-5 seeds.
- Greenish gray or gray in colour, flat (disk-shaped), the testa is hairy, odorless with very bitter taste.

4. Nux Vomica Seeds

o Origin: East India (Tropical regions).

Constituents:

Alkaloids (strychnine, brucine).

Chemical tests:

The thin sections of nuxvomica seed are defatted and the following tests are performed.

1. Stain the transverse section of nuxvomica with ammonium vanadate and sulphuric acid (Manddin's reagent). The endospermic cells become purple due to the presence of strychnine.
2. Stain the transverse section of nuxvomica with concentrated nitric acid. Endospermic cells take yellow colour due to the presence of brucine.
3. Strychnine with sulphuric acid and potassium dichromate gives violet colour which turns to red and finally yellow.

Uses:

Very toxic plant, appetite stimulant in small doses.

Adulterants:

It is found to be adulterated with dried seeds of *Strychnos nuxblanda* and *Strychnos potatorum*.

Substitute:

The seeds of *Strychnos wallichiana* are used as substitute.

4. Nux Vomica Seeds

Microscopical characters:

Testa:

Hairy epidermis:

Single layered; each epidermal cell forms a lignified trichomes comprising of a pitted bulbous base and a projection which is narrowly elongated and slightly bent beyond the base. The trichomes of all epidermal cells run parallel in one direction giving the testa of the seed a silky appearance. Collapsed parenchyma: Two layered collapsed parenchymatous cells with yellowish brown contents.

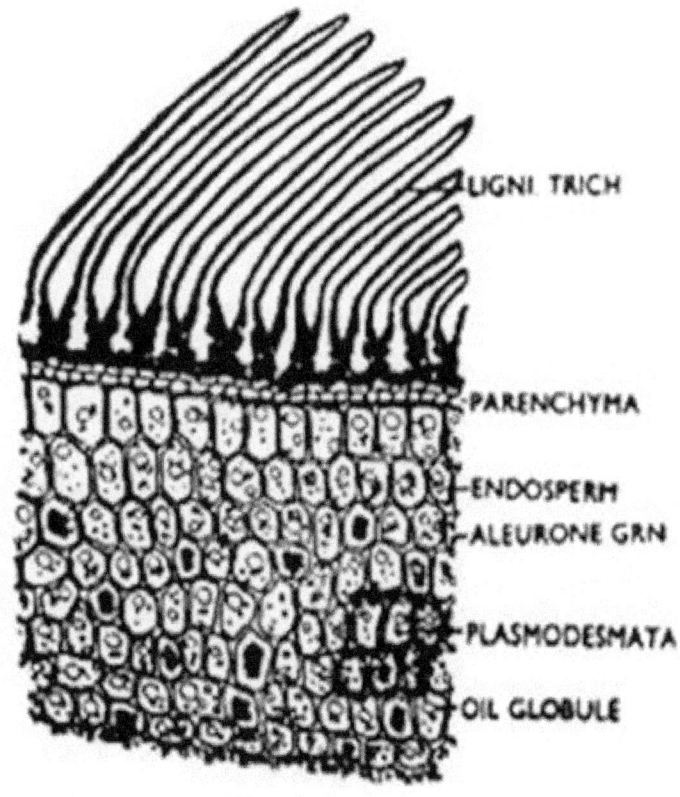

4. Nux Vomica Seeds

Endosperm:
They form the bulk of the seed. Outermost layers of the endosperm below the collapsed parenchyma appear palisade like whereas the inner layers contain cells which are polyhedral. The cells of endosperm also contain aleurone grains and oil droplets.

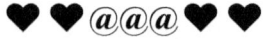

5. SENNA LEAVES:
SENNA LEAFLETS: FOLIA SENNAE

Latin names:

Cassia acutifolia Vahl. Synonym Cassia senna L.- (Alexandrian Senna or Egyptian Senna)

Cassia angustifolia Vahl. – (Indian Senna or Tinnevelly senna)

Family: *Leguminosae*

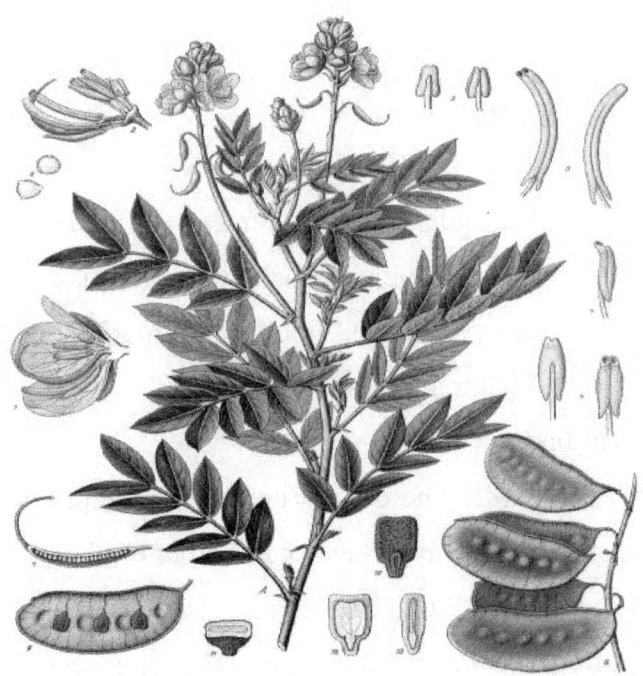

Cassia acutifolia

Notes: ***Cassia acutifolia***: the leaves with acute apex

Cassia angustifolia*:* plant with narrow leaves

- Perennial small trees (shrubs).

5. Senna Leaves

- Fruits form: legume with 3-5 seeds (dark brown).
- Leaves are small & dark green, but after drying turn yellow.
- Colour: dry leaves yellowish green.
- Odour: distinctive, not penetrating.
- Taste: first slimy sweetish, later bitter and harsh.
- Origin: Mecca then cultivated in Egypt, Sudan & India.

Chemical constituents:
1. Glycosides: Anthraquinone group:
   Sennoside A & B, and traces of C & D.
2. Resins, Flavone derivatives (yellow).
3. Rhein & Aloe emodin Anthraquinone (free anthraquinone).

Chemical test:

Borntrager's test: The drug is boiled with sulphuric acid, filtered and to the filtrate, benzene or ether or chloroform is added and shaken well. The organic layer is separated to which ammonia is added slowly. The ammonical layer shows pink to red colour due to presence of anthraquinone glycosides.

5. Senna Leaves

Uses

Treatment of constipation. In small doses laxative, but in large doses purgative.

Adulterants:

It is found to be adulterated with Dog senna (*C. obovata*), Palthe senna (*C. auriculata*) and Mumbai, Mecca and Arabian senna.

Microscopical examination:

The characteristic key elements are:

- The leaves hair (b1, d).
- Paracytic stoma (g).
- Calcium oxalate druses (c).
- Sclerenchyma fibers (vascular tissue with crystals) (f).
- Mucilaginous cell (e).

a) Fragment with a leaf cross section, upper palisade parenchyma (1), spongy parenchyma with Ca-oxalate (2), lower palisade parenchyma (3).

b 1) epidermal fragment with hair.

b 2) epidermal fragment with broken hair.

c) Calcium oxalate druses.

d) Broken hair.

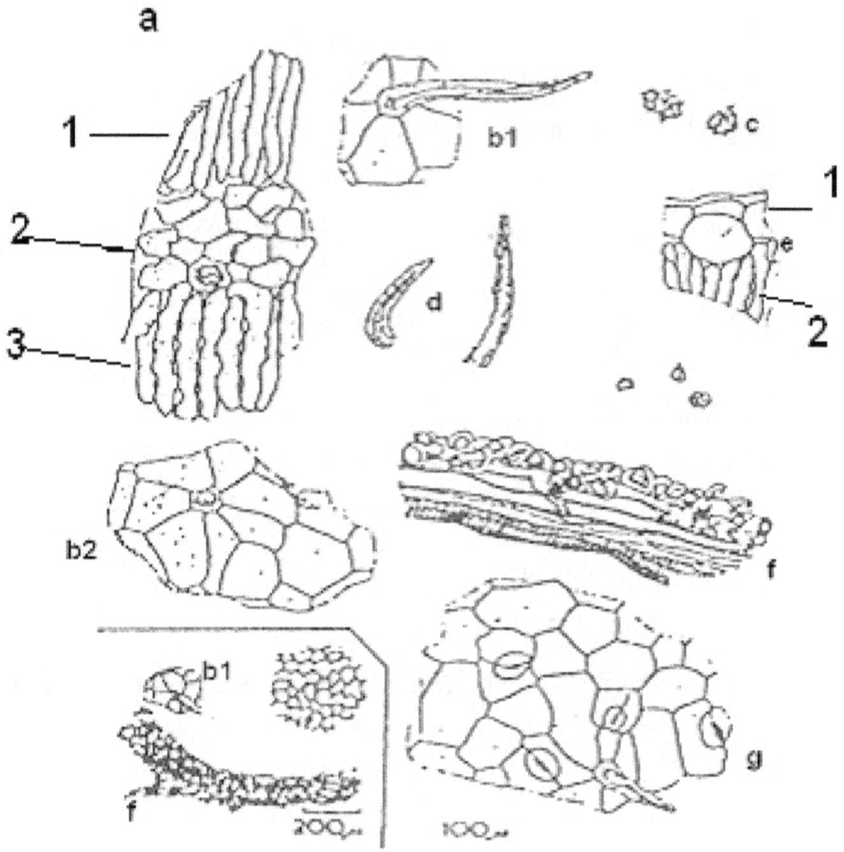

5. Senna Leaves

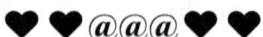

e) Fragment of mucilagenous cell between epidermises (1) and palisade parenchyma (2).

f) Fragment of schelernchyma fibers.

g) Epidermal fragment with paracytic stomata.

♥ ♥ @@@ ♥ ♥

6. RHUBARB RHIZOMES: RADIX RHEI

Synonyms: Radix rhei, Rheum, Revandchini.

Latin name: *Rheum officinale* or *Rheum rhaponticum L.* (Japanese Rhubarb)

Rheum palmatum S.L. (Chinese Rhubarb)

Family: *Polygonaceae*

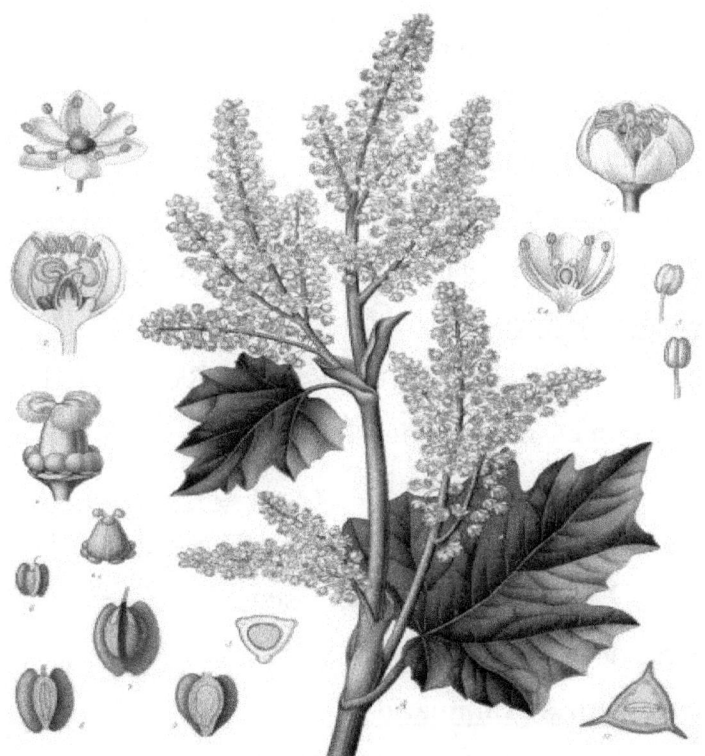

Rheum officinale

- ✓ Perennial trees with large roots and rhizomes.
- ✓ Colour: pale brown or brown color.

6. Rhubarb Rhizomes

- Odourless.
- Taste: astringent and bitter.
- Origin : China, Japan.
- **Chemical constituent** :
- 1. Anthraquinone. (Free State).
    a. emodin anthraquinone.
    b. aloe emodine anthraquinone.
    c. rhein anthraquinone.
    d. rhein anthrones.
    e. chrysophanol anthraquinones.
  2. Tannins:
    a. Gallic acid (pseudo tannin).
    b. Glucogallin (true tannin hydrolysable group).

Identification test:

Test for anthraquinone (Brontrager test); Powder + H_2O + KOH → intensive red colour.

Uses:

In small doses = 1g → stomachic, antidiarrheal, astringent and haemostatic.

In large doses > 1-3 g → purgative.

Microscopical examination

The characteristic key elements are:

1. Calcium oxalate druses (a).
2. Pitted reticular vessels(c).

6. Rhubarb Rhizomes

3. Elongated or rounded –polygonal, thin-walled parenchyma cells.

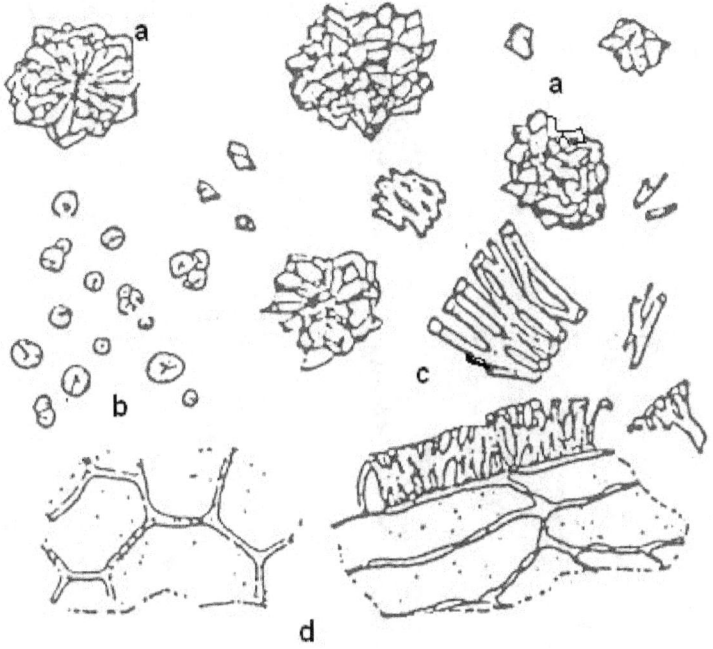

a) Calcium oxalate druses & their fragments
b) Starch grains
c) Fragments of very wide, coarsely pitted reticular vessels

(No wood reaction with phloroglucin hydrochloric acid)

d) Fragments from the parenchyma, elongated or rounded –polygonal, thin-walled cells, frequently with many starch grains.

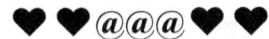

7. DIGITALIS LEAVES:
FOXGLOVE LEAVES: FOLIA DIGITALI

Latin names: *Digitalis purpurea L.; Digitalis lanata L*
Family: *Scrophulariaceae*

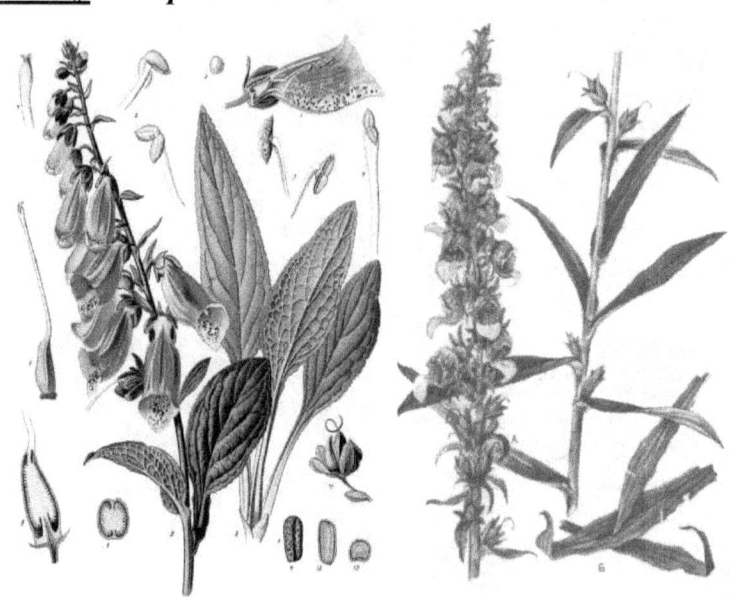

| D. purpurea | D. lanata |

Biennial or perennial herbaceous plant reaches 1-1.5 meters in height with bell-shaped flowers.

Both leaves surfaces are hairy.

D.Purpurea: has hairy leaves with purple flowers.

D.Lanata: has very hairy leaves with whitish pink flowers.

Colour: dark grayish green

Odour: no marked odour.

Taste: distinctly bitter.

7. Digitalis Leaves

Origin:

Southern and Central regions of Europe.

Chemical constituents

Glycosides: cardiac (steroidal) group:

1. Digoxin.
2. Digitoxin.
3. Gitoxin.

Chemical tests:

Keller-Kiliani test for digitoxose: The test consists of boiling about 1 g finely powdered digitalis with 10 ml 70% alcohol for 2 to 3 minutes. The extract is filtered. To the filtrate is added, 5 ml water and 0.5 ml strong solution of lead acetate. Shake well and separate the filtrate. The clear filtrate is treated with equal volume of chloroform and evaporated to yield the extractive. The extractive is dissolved in glacial acetic acid and after cooling, 2 drops ferric chloride solution are added to it. These contents are transferred to a test tube containing 2 ml concentrated sulphuric acid. A reddish brown layer acquiring bluish-green colour after standing is observed due to the presence of digitoxose.

Legal test: The extract is dissolved in pyridine, sodium nitroprusside solution is added to it and made alkaline-pink or red colour is produced.

7. Digitalis Leaves

Baljet test: To a section of digitalis, sodium picrate solution is added. It shows yellow to orange colour.

Uses
1. Congestive heart failure.
2. Arrhythmia.

Adulterants:

Digitalis leaves are adulterated with the leaves of *Verbascum thapsus* (Scrophulariaceae), *Primula vulgaris* (Primulaceae) and *Symphytum officinale* (Boraginaceae).

Microscopical examinations:

Characteristic microscopical features:
1. Anomocytic stoma (2).
2. Covering trichome (4).
3. Trichome with a collapsed cell (10).
4. Glandular trichomes with unicellular heads (11).
5. Fragment of a large covering trichomes (13).
6. Epidermis in sectional view showing pitting in the walls and a glandular trichome.
7. Fragments of covering trichomes. (a) Apical cell and (b) Basal cell attached to a fragment of epidermis.
8. Cortical parenchyma in longitudinal view.
9. Epidermis in surface view showing cicatrices.

7. Digitalis Leaves

10. Part of a covering trichomes showing a collapsed cell.

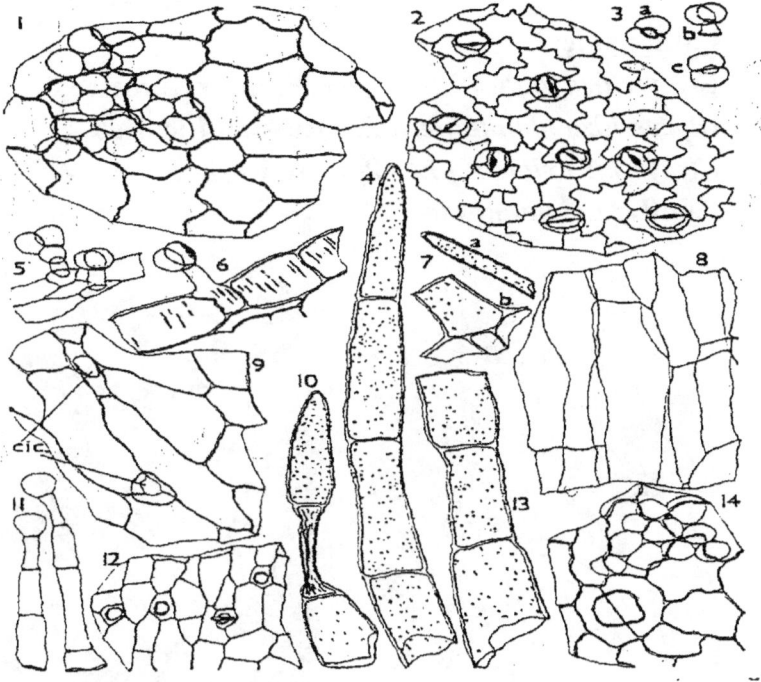

11. Glandular trichome with uniseriate stalks and unicellular heads.

12. Epidermis from over a vein in surface view showing cicatrices.

13. Fragment of a large covering trichomes.

14. Upper epidermis in surface view showing a cicatrix and underlying palisade cells.

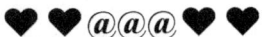

8. LIQUORICE:
GLYCYRRHIZA: SWEET ROOTS: RADIX LIQUIRITIAE

Latin name:
Glycyrrhiza glabra L. -English, Spanish Licorice;
Glycyrrhiza glandulifera L. - Russian Licorice
Glycyrrhiza violacea L. - Persian Licorice
Family: *Leguminosae*

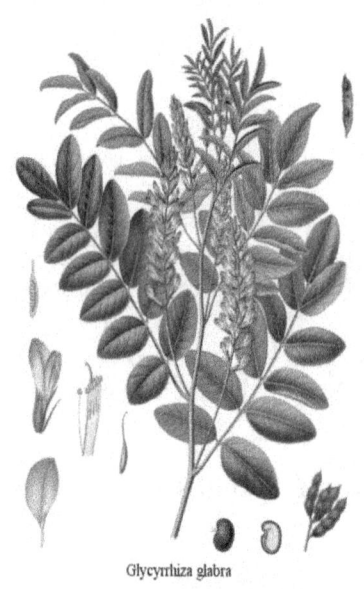

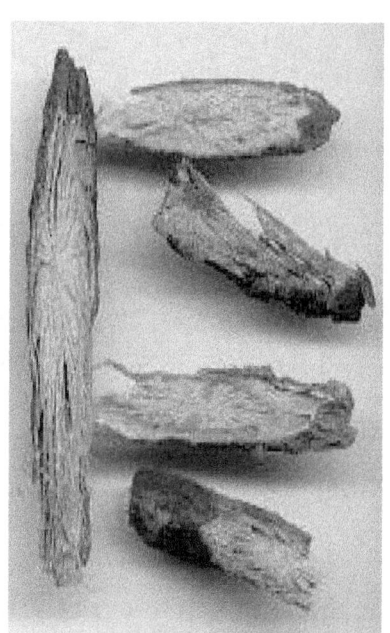

Fresh Licorice roots

- Perennial small trees.
- Fruit form legume.
- Colour: the roots outer surface brown or reddish brown while inner surface yellowish brown.
- Odor: weak, somewhat aromatic.

8. Liquorice

- Taste: sweet.

Chemical constituents
1. Glycoside –Saponin group: Glycyrrhizin 50 times sweeter than sucrose.
2. Flavonoids –Liquiritin & Isoliquiritin.
3. Proteins.
4. Sugars (glucose, sucrose).

Chemical test:
On addition of 0% sulphuric acid, the thick section of drug or powder shows deep yellow colour.

Uses:
1. Expectorant.
2. Antihistaminic.
3. Flavoring agent for Aloe, Quinine, NH_4CL, Chocolates.
4. Anti-inflammatory activity –used in treatment of peptic ulcer seborrhea & mucous membranes ulcers.
5. Demulcent.
6. Soft drink.

8. Liquorice

Adulterants and substitutes:

Manchurian liquorice obtained from *Glycyrrhiza uralensis*. Russian liquorice may be peeled and obtained from *Glycyrrhiza glabra* variety *glandulifera*.

Microscopical examination

Key elements:

1. Sclerenchymal fibers (c).
2. Reticular vessels (d).
3. Cortical parenchyma (f).
4. Fragments from the pith with crystal cell layers (b).

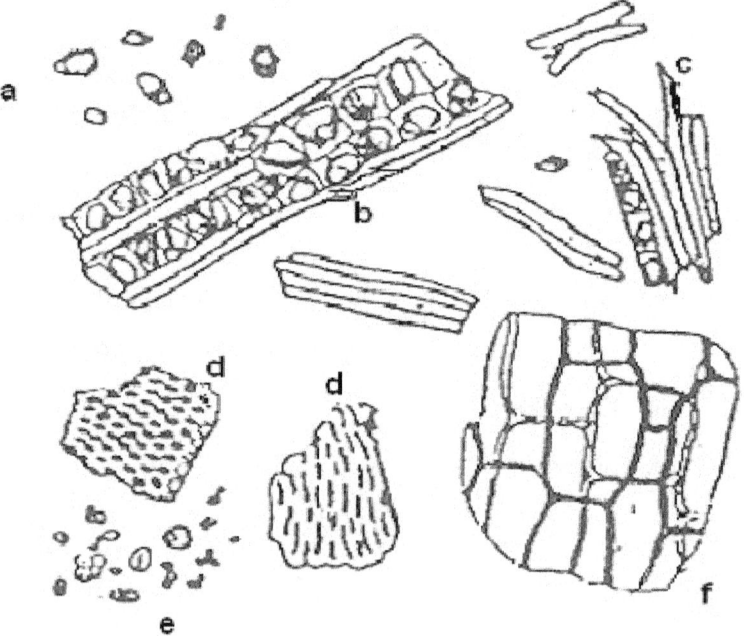

8. Liquorice

a) Ca-oxalate single crystals from the crystal cell layers.
b) Fragments from the pith with crystal cell layers & subjacent yellowish sclerenchymal fibers.
c) Sclerenchymal fiber fragments.
d) Yellowish fragments of often very wide vessels with pit zones & areola thickened walls.
e) Starch particles from the cortical & wood parenchyma of rounded or spindle to rod shape.
f) Fragments of cells from cortical parenchyma.

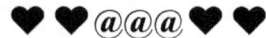

9. FENUGREEK SEED: SEMIN TRIGONELLAE

Latin name: *Trigonella foenum graecum L.*

Family: *Leguminosae*

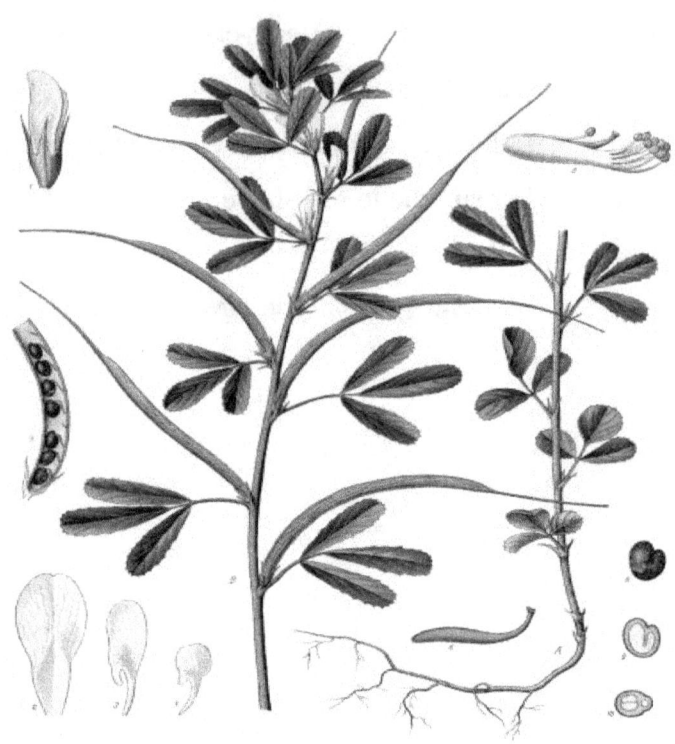

Trigonella foenum graecum L.
- Annual herbaceous plant
- Yellow or pale brown, or dark yellow (coloured seed)
- Odor: characteristics (aromatic).
- Taste : bitter taste
- Origin: Mediterranean Sea region (Greece).

9. Fenugreek Seed

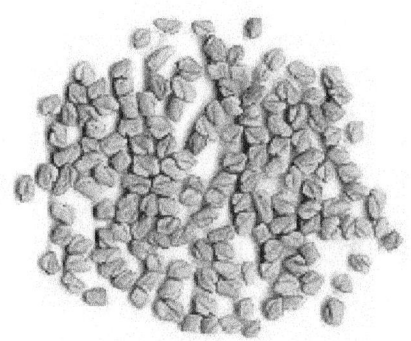

Fenugreek seeds

Chemical constituents:

1. Saponin glycoside.
2. Fixed oil 66%.
3. Protein.
4. Mucilage.
5. Alkaloids (trigonilline, choline).
6. Bitter principles.
7. Phytosteroids

Uses:

1. Nutrient.
2. Demulcent.
3. Lactogenic.
4. Stomachic.
5. Hypoglycemic agent.
6. U.T. antiseptic

Microscopical examination

9. Fenugreek Seed

The characteristic key elements:
1. Epidermis of the testa (a).
2. Corona- (cuticle, epidermis, hypodermis of the testa) (b).
3. Hypodermis of the testa (c).
4. Epidermis & paranchymatous cells of the cotyledons (e).

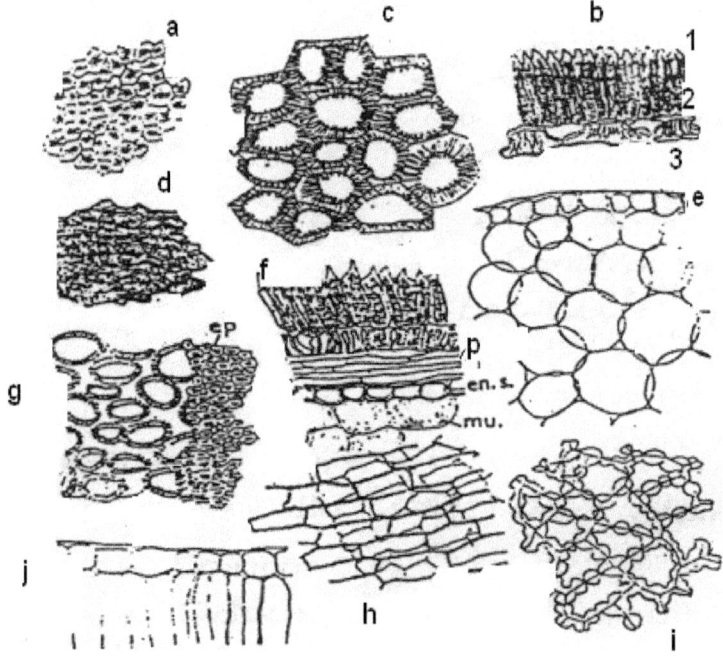

a) Epidermis of the testa in top view
b) Cuticle (1), epidermis (2), hypodermis (3) of the testa in sectional view
c) Hypodermis of the testa in surface view from below
d) Epidermis of the testa in surface view from below

9. Fenugreek Seed

e) Epidermis & paranchymatous cells of the cotyledons in sectional view

f) Part of the seed in sectional view showing the epidermis, hypodermis, paranchymatous layer (p) of the testa & the outermost layer (en.s) & the mucilage cells (mu) of the endosperm

g) Epidermis (ep) & hypodermis of the testa in top view

h) Layers of the parenchyma of the testa in surface view

i) Outermost layer of the endosperm in surface view

j) Epidermis & palisade of the cotyledons in sectional view

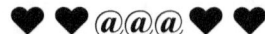

10. LINSEED (FLAX SEED): SEMIN LINI

Latin name: *Linum usitatissimum L.*

Family: *Linaceae*

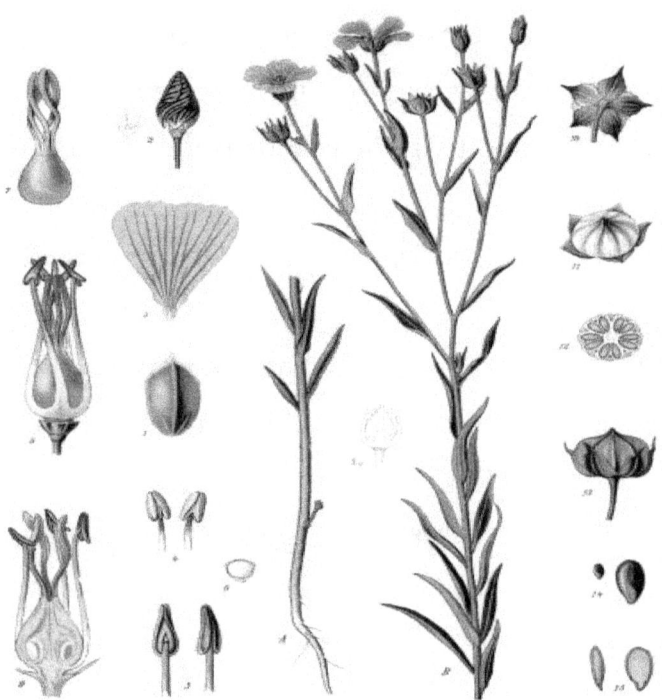

Linum usitatissimum L.

- Annual herbaceous plant, with blue flowers.
- Colour: pale brown coloured seeds.
- Odourless.
- Taste: mucilagenous taste (Nutty).
- Origin: tropical regions.

10. Linseed (Flax Seed)

Chemical constituents:

1- Fixed oil 30-40 % (Lin oil).

2- Protein (in aleurone layer).

3- Mucilage.

4- Cyanogenic glycoside (linmarin).

Uses of linseed oil:

1. Demulcent.

2. Mild laxative.

3. Emollient.

4. Cosmetics (creams and lotions).

5. Industrial uses (paint & varnishes "drying oil", ink and soap.

Microscopical examination:

Characteristic microscopical features:

1. Pigment cell layer (b).
2. Fragment from the seed coat (c).
3. Cotyledon tissue (e).

10. Linseed (Flax Seed)

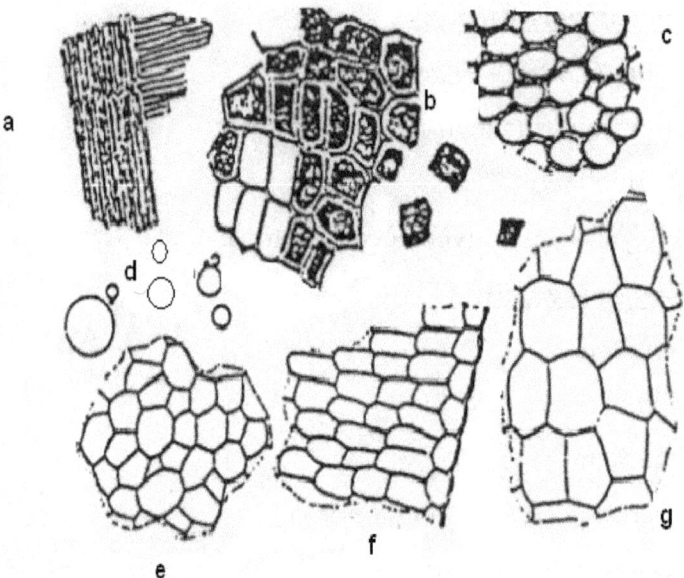

a) Fragment of internal integument with the cells of the sclerenchymal fiber layer, cells from the peripendicular layer
b) Fragment from the pigment cell layer and pigment aggregates in top view
c) Fragment from the seed coat in top view
d) Oil droplets
e) Fragment from the cotyledon tissue
f) Fragment from the cotyledon in cross section
g) Fragment from the seed coat epidermis in top view

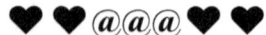

11. BLACK MUSTARD SEEDS: SINAPIS NIGRAE SEMINA

Latin name: *Brassica nigra L.*
Family: *Cruciferae*

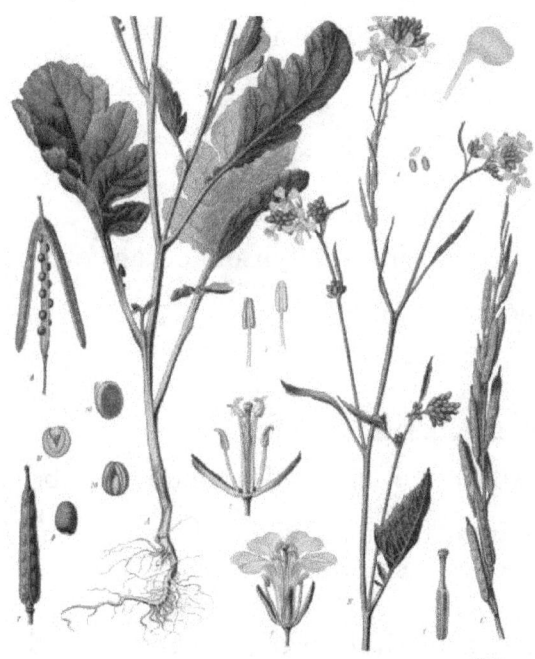

Brassica nigra L

- ✓ Annual herbaceous plant with yellow flowers and cruciferous leaves.
- ✓ The seeds are globular, the testa is dark reddish-brown to yellow.
- ✓ The embryo is oily and greenish-yellow or yellow in colour.

11. Black Mustard Seeds

- Taste: pungent.
- Odour: characteristic.
- Origin: Europe and south western of Asia and cultivated in temperate regions.

Chemical constituents:

1- Thiocyanate glycosides (sinigrin) 0.7-1.3%.

2- Enzyme myrosin.

3- Fixed oil 27%.

4- Proteins 30%.

Sinigrin (by myrosin) → allylisothiocyanate (mustard oil, V.O) + glucose + $KHSO_4$.

Test for Black Mustard seeds:

Powdered Black Mustard seeds acquire much brighter yellow colour on treatment with Alkali solution.

Uses:

Condiment, emetic (if the dose > 10 gm), rubefacient, counter irritant and stomachic.

Microscopical examination

Characteristic key elements:

1. Mucilaginous epidermis of the testa & sclereids (a).
2. Aleurone & oil droplets (c).
3. Thin walled epidermis filled with mucilage (e).

11. Black Mustard Seeds

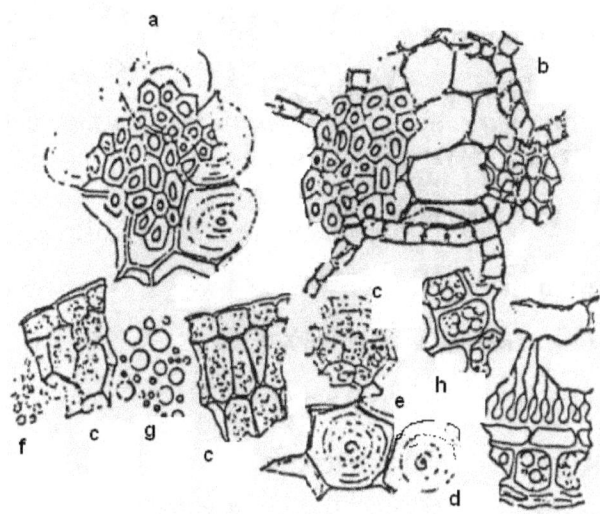

a) Fragments of mucilaginous epidermis of the testa & sclereids in surface view
b) Fragments of sclereids & the parenchyma (pigmented) of the embryo parenchyma
c) Aleurone & oil droplets of the embryo parenchyma
d) Fragments of the testa in T.S with mucilaginous epidermis sclereids & oil droplets.
e) Thin walled epidermis filled with mucilage
f) Well-formed aleurone grains with crystalloid & globoid
g) Oil droplets
h) Fragments of polygonal cells filled with oil droplets.

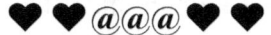

12. CINNAMON BARK: CORTEX CINNAMOMI

Latin name: *Cinnamomum zeylanicum Nees.* (Ceylon Cinnamon) (Sri Lanka)

Cinnamomum cassia Nees. (Chinese Cinnamon)

Family: *Lauraceae*

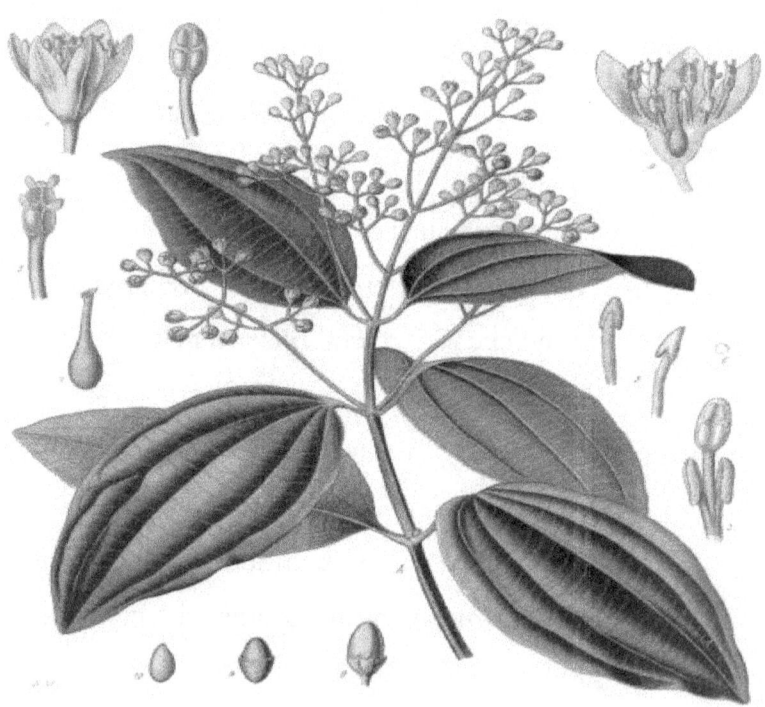

Cinnamomum cassia

- Perennial handsome evergreen large trees.
- The bark external surface: dark brown.
- The bark inner surface yellowish brown.

12. Cinnamon Bark

- Odor: aromatic.
- Taste: warm, sweet and aromatic.
- Origin: Sri Lanka & China.

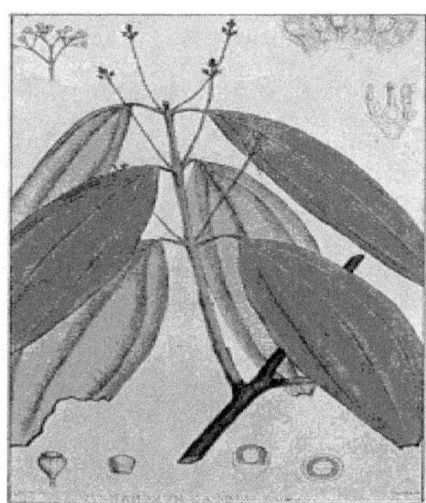
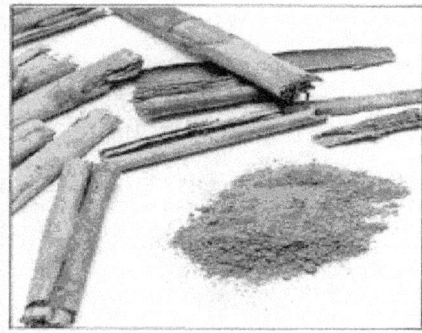

Cinnamon
Cinamomum cassia

Chemical constituents

C. zeylanicum constituents:

1. Cinnamon oil (volatile oil):
   a. Cinnamic aldehyde 60-70%.
   b. Eugenol.
2. Mucilage (Mannitol)
3. Sugars
4. Starch.
5. Tannins (phlobatannin).

Cinnamon cassia has the same constituents except eugenol.

12. Cinnamon Bark

Contains Cinnamic aldehyde 80%.

Chemical test:

On addition of a drop of ferric chloride solution to a drop of volatile oil, a pale green colour is produced. With ferric chloride, cinnamic aldehyde gives brown colour and eugenol gives blue colour, resulting in the formation of pale green colour.

In cassia oil, brown colour is obtained, as it contains only cinnamic aldehyde.

Uses
1. Carminative.
2. Flavor.
3. Antiseptic.
4. Antidiarrhea.
5. Powerful germicide.

Substitutes and adulterants:
1. Jungle cinnamon
2. Cinnamon chips
3. Saigon cinnamon (*Cinnamomum loureirii*)
4. Java cinnamon (*Cinnamomum burmanii*)

12. Cinnamon Bark

Microscopical examination

Key elements:

1. Modularly ray tissue with calcium oxalate needles (a).
2. Fibers (b).
3. Stone cells (c).

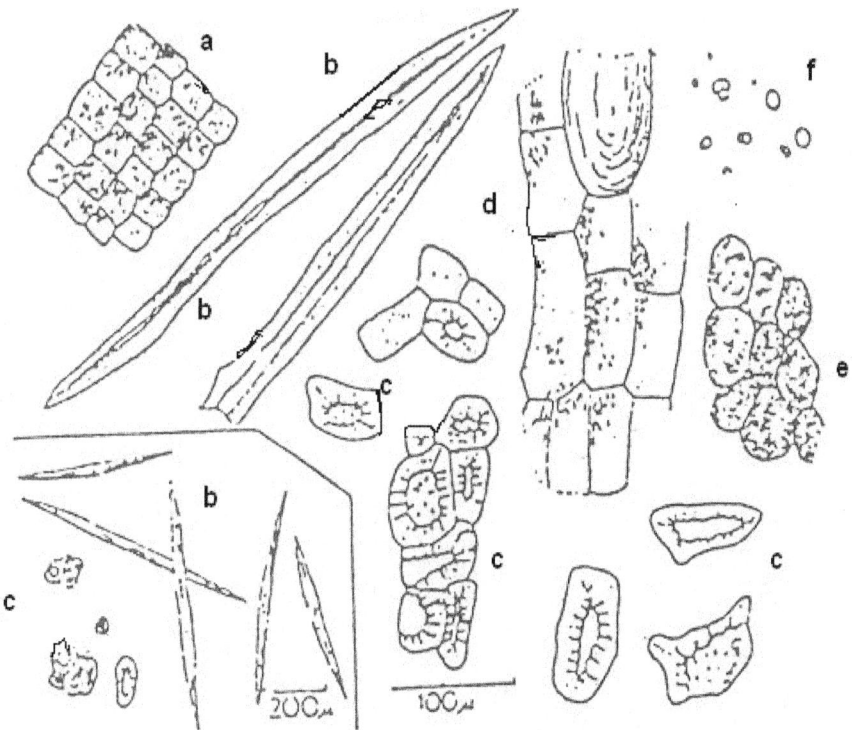

a) Cells of modularly ray tissue with calcium oxalate needles.
b) Fibers & fiber fragments.
c) Stone cells from primary bark.

12. Cinnamon Bark

d) Cells from the cortical parenchyma with crystal needles and occluded excretory cell.

e) Cells from cortical parenchyma.

f) Starch grains.

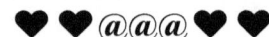

13. CLOVE BUDS: FLOS CARYOPHYLLI

Latin name: *Eugenia caryophyllus* (Sprengel) or *Eugenia caryophyllata* (Thunberg)

Family: *Myrtaceae*

- Perennial large trees (15) m height.
- The buds collected when their colour changed from green to red.
- Dried clove buds colour: reddish brown.
- Taste: pungent & acrid.
- Odor: aromatic like the odor of Pepper and Cinnamon together.
- Origin: Madagascar & Sumatra.

Chemical constituents:

1. Volatile oil (Clove oil) 14%-20%.
A. Eugenol 70%-90%.
B. Vanillin.
C. Caryophyllene 1%.
D. Acetyl eugenol 4%.
2. Tannin: Gallotannic acid 10-13%.

13. Clove Buds

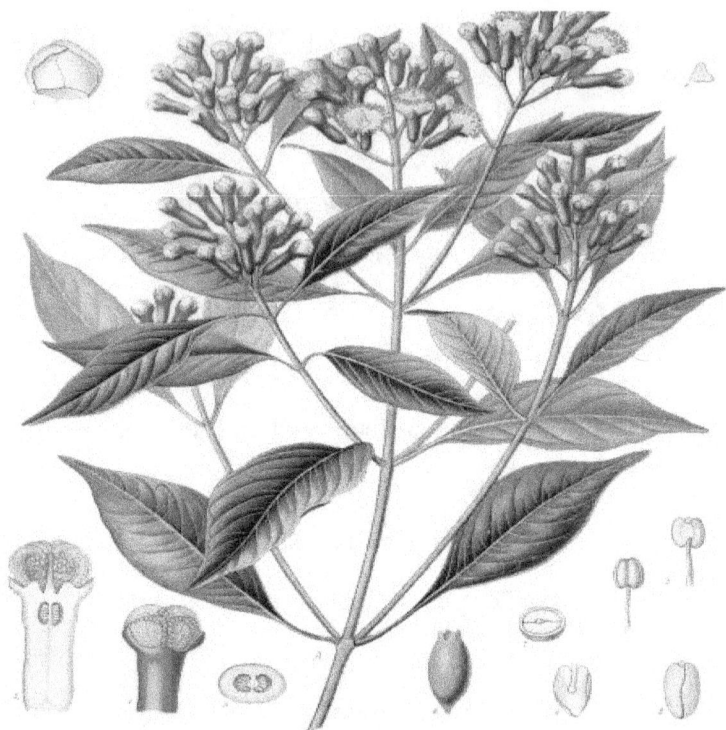

Eugenia caryophyllus

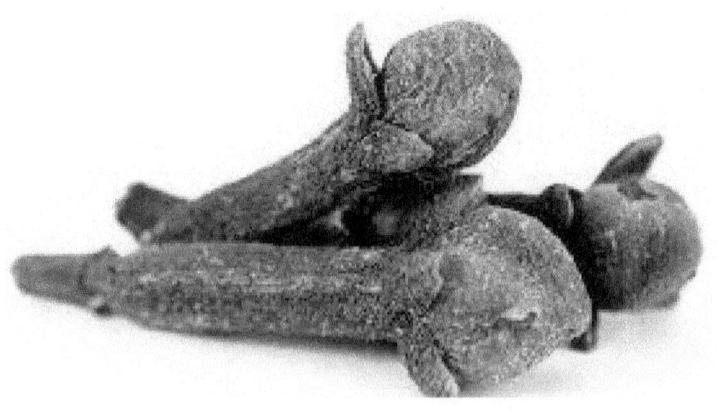

13. Clove Buds

Chemical test:

If the transverse section of clove is treated with strong potassium hydroxide solution, the needle shaped crystals of potassium eugenate are observed.

Uses:
1. Condiment.
2. Carminative.
3. Clove oil which contains high percentage of eugenol used commercially to produce Vanillin.
4. Antiseptic.
5. Flavoring agent.
6. Dental uses: as filling material with ZnO.
7. Local anesthetic (dental analgesic).

Adulterants:
1. Mother cloves
2. Brown cloves
3. Clove stalks
4. Exhausted cloves

Microscopical examination

Characteristic microscopical features:
1. Sclerenchymatose fiber from the bud (f).
2. Secretory glands (b2).
3. Pollen grains with 3 emergences(C).

13. Clove Buds

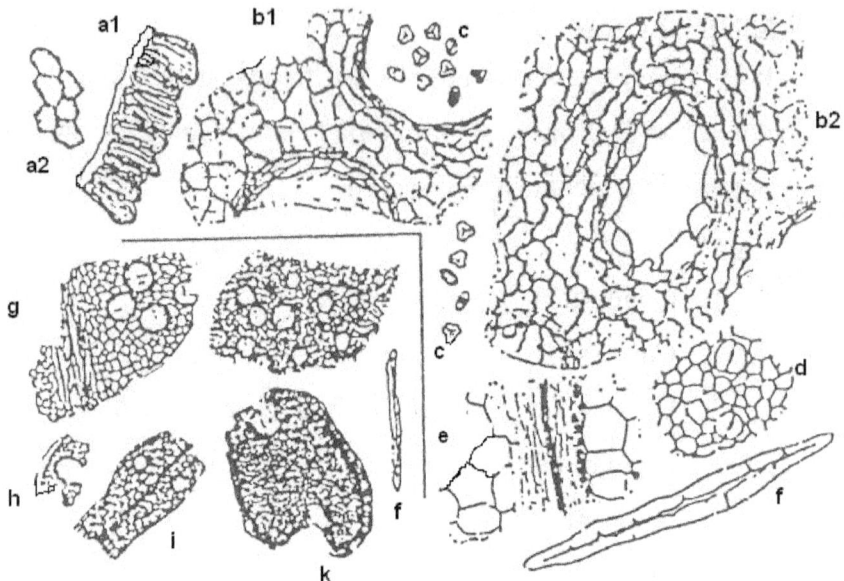

a1) Anther fragment in side view 1. Epidermis 2. Fiber cells.

a2) Anther fragment, fiber cells of anther in top view.

b1, b2) Fragments from the bud parenchyma with secretory glands (b2) & residues of
   two Secretory glands (b1) in the center of (b2).

c) Pollen grains with 3 emergences.

d) Epidermis fragment with 2 large somatal apertures in top view.

e) Tissue fragment from the bud with vascular bundle & neighboring crystal cell
   layer.

f) Schlerenchyma fiber from the bud.

13. Clove Buds

g) Tissue fragment with numerous secretory glands & vessels, left fragment with
  schlerenchyma fibers.

h) Fragment from the bud wall, residue from a secretory gland.

i) Style fragment with central vascular bundle & 2 secretory glands.

k) Anther (torn) with numerous pollen grains in the interior.

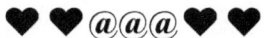

14. GINGER RHIZOME: JAMAICA GINGER: RHIZOMA ZINGIBERIS

Latin name: *Zingiber officinalis   Rosco.*

Family: *Zingiberaceae*

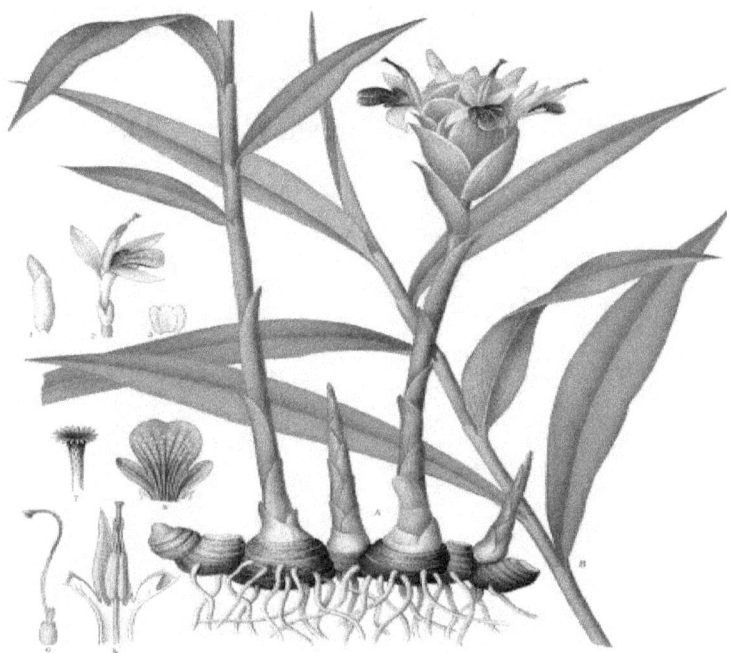

Zingiber officinale

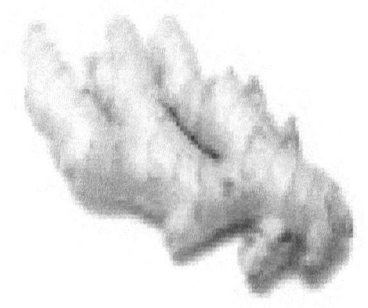

14. Ginger Rhizome

Fresh Ginger rhizome

- Perennial herbaceous plant with large leaves.
- Colour: brown or pale brown.
- Odor: aromatic.
- Taste: pungent and acrid.
- Origin : Africa, India and Central America.

Chemical constituents:

1. Volatile oil 3% (zingiberene, zingiberol, zingiberenol, zingerone).
2. Starch 50 %.
3. Protein.
4. Sugars (glucose, sucrose).
5. Resins (oleo- resin).

Uses:

Carminative, condiment, flavouring agent, cause anorexia, popular drink.

Used also in the throat problems (voice loss).

Adulterant:

Ginger is adulterated with exhausted ginger.

Microscopical examination

The characteristic key elements are:

1. Starch granules (50%) (e).
2. Scalar form vessel (a).
3. Sclerenchymal fiber (b).

14. Ginger Rhizome

4. Parenchyma & oleo-resin cell (d).

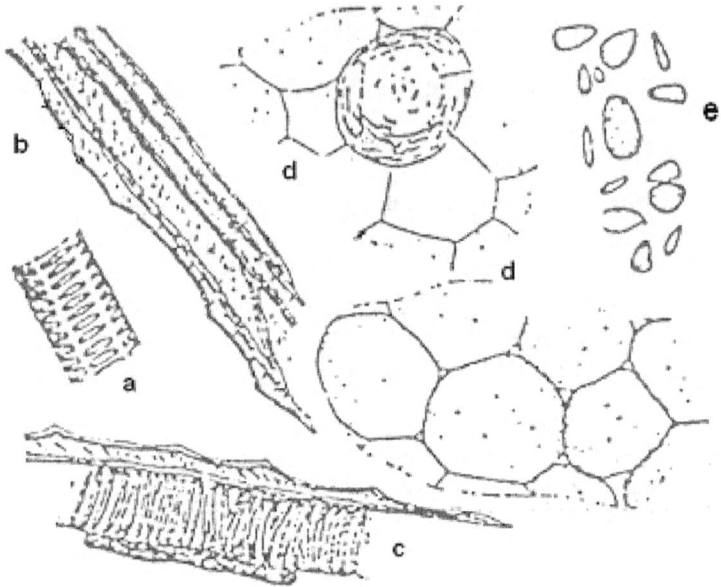

a) Fragment of a scalar vessel.
b) Fragment of broken sclerenchymal fiber from a vascular bundle, cell walls slightly thickened, pits oblique & slit shaped.
c) Vessel fragment with adjoining sclerenchymal fibers (top, see also b) & elongated oil cells (bottom).
d) Parenchyma & oleo-resin cell.
e) Starch granules, more or less flattened with end protruberance (usually at the narrower end), stratification present in most cases.

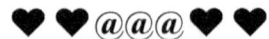

15. CHAMOMILE FLOWERS (FLOS CHAMOMILLAE)

Latin name: *Matricaria chamomilla L.*-German chamomile

Family: *Compositae*

Other species:

1- *Anthemis cotula*

2- *Anthemis arvensis*

3- *Anthemis nobilis* –Roman Chamomile.

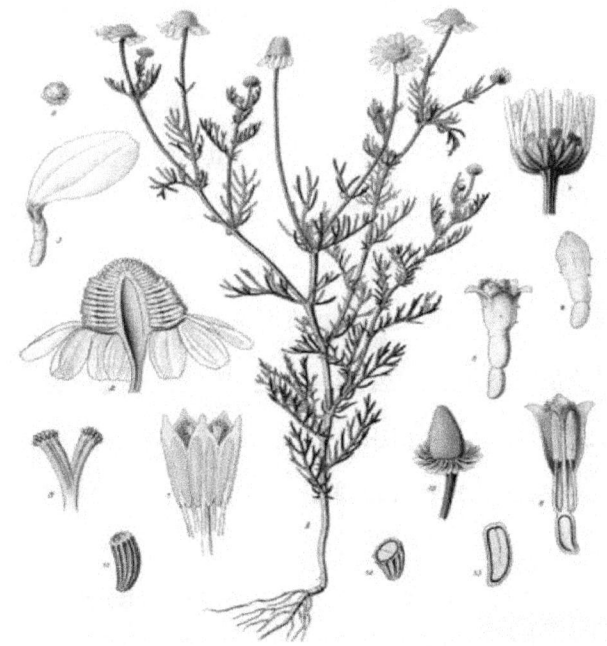

Matricaria chamomilla L.-German chamomile

15. Chamomile Flowers

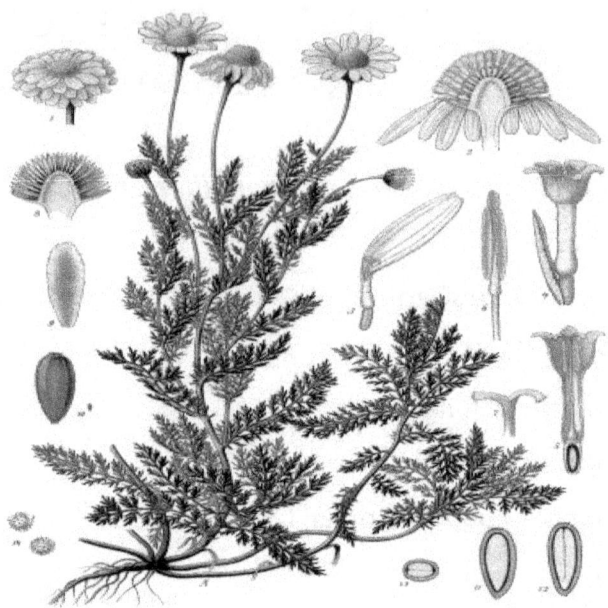

Anthemis nobilis

- Perennial herbaceous plant with white flowers.

Odor: aromatic.

Taste: slight bitter.

Origin: Mediterranean regions, Europe.

Roman Chamomile is not so rich in volatile oils like German Chamomile

Chemical constituents

1. Volatile oil (1%) Chamomile oil:
   a) Azulene (chamazulene)-sesqueterpenes.
   b) Bisabolol.
2. Bitter principles: anthemic acid.
3. Flavonoids (apigenin – a trihydroxy flavone).

15. Chamomile Flowers

Uses:
1. Antispasmodic.
2. Antiseptic.
3. Anti-inflammatory (respiratory system {vapor inhalations}) inflammations & ophthalmic inflammations.
4. Carminative.
5. Stomachic.
6. Cosmetics (facial creams, skin lotions, shampoo).
7. Diuretic.

Microscopical examination for German Chamomile:
Characteristic microscopical features:
1. Petal tips from a disk (a).
2. Connective of a stamen (b).
3. Pollen grains (f).
4. Side of stigma (j).
5. Stone cells from the base of the ovary (g).

a) Petal tip from a disk (upper epidermis in top view), elongated epidermis cells, more or less rectangular, cell walls sometimes more or less undulated.

b) Connective of a stamen.

c) Epidermis cells with compositae gland in top view.

15. Chamomile Flowers

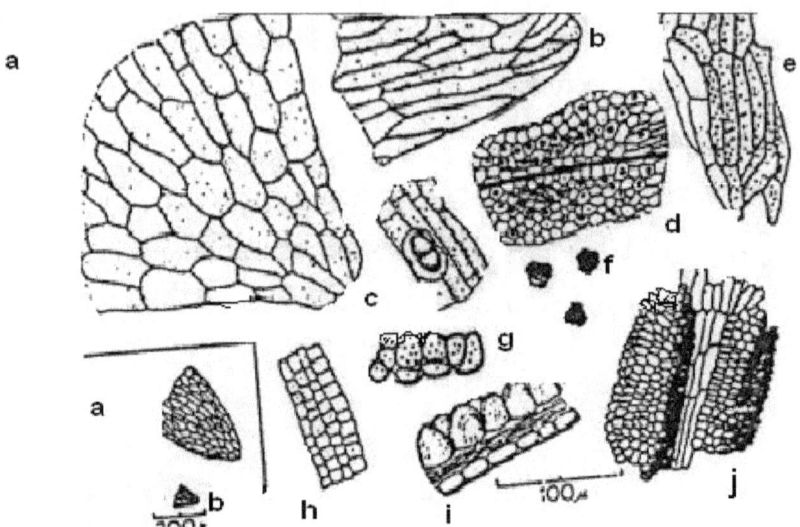

c) Fragment of a petal in top view, mesophyll cells with small Ca-oxalate rosettes.
d) Fragment from the sepal, greenish cell wall at times sclerenchymatose & pitted.
e) Pollen grains with granular echinate structure & 3 emergences.
f) Stone cells from the base of the ovary.
g) Fragment from the filament epidermis in top view, filament thin, rounded with central vascular bundle.
h) Epidermis fragment from the petal of a ray, outer wall of inner epidermis. strikingly papillose, cuticle striation.
i) Side of stigma.

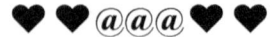

16. FRUCTUS ANISI: ANISE FRUIT

Latin name: *Pimpinella anisum L.*

Family: *Umbelliferae*

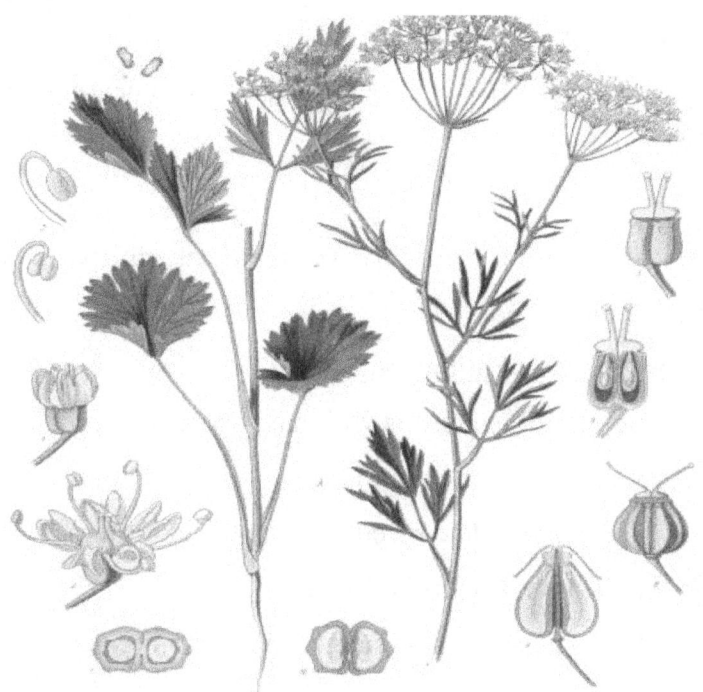

Pimpinella anisum

- Annual herbaceous plant, with white flowers.
- Fruit form cremocarp with 5 primary ridges.
- Colour: pale brown to green seeds.
- Odour: aromatic (typical anethole odor).
- Taste: sweet aromatic.
- Origin: Egypt and Europe.

16. Fructus Anisi

Chemical constituents:
1. Volatile oil (Anethole 90%, chavicol).
2. Fixed oil.
3. Protein.

Identification of volatile oil:

Powder + Sudan III → red oil droplets (with heating oil droplets remain)

Uses:

Carminative, popular drink, flavoring agent, antispasmodic and condiment.

Microscopical examination:
1. Seed wall epidermis with hairs (arcuate hairs, verrucose hair cuticle) (a).
2. Calcium oxalate rosettes from the endosperm indication for Umbelliferae seeds(e).
3. Endosperm with minute calcium oxalate rosettes (h).
4. Fragment of the seed wall epidermis with hairs (arcuate hairs, verrucose hair cuticle).
5. Fragment of seed wall epidermis.
6. c1) Tissue fragments with yellow- brown secretary ducts, epithelial cells, and transverse cells.
   c2) like c1 but without epithelial cells.

16. Fructus Anisi

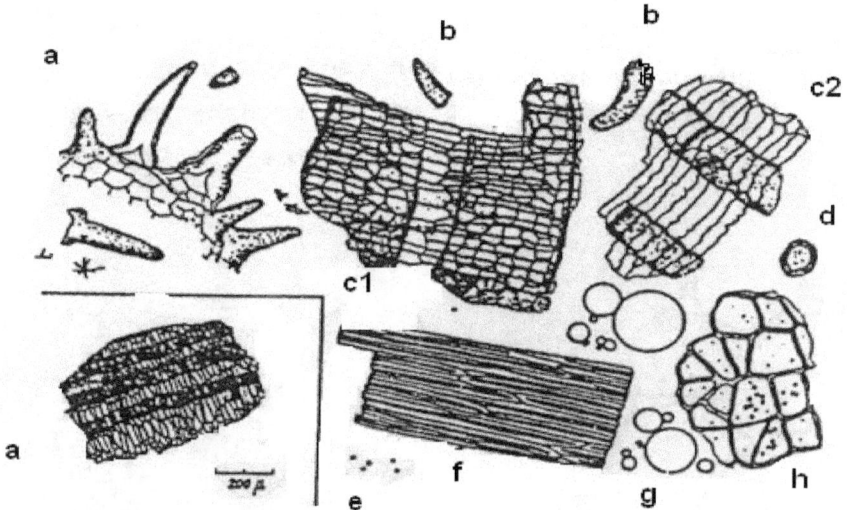

d) Stone cells.

e) Calcium oxalate rosettes from the endosperm indication for Umbelliferae seeds.

f) Sclerenchymal fibers.

g) Droplet of fatty oil.

h) Fragments from the endosperm with minute calcium oxalate rosettes.

♥ ♥ @@@ ♥ ♥

17. CARAWAY FRUITS

Latin name: *Carum carvi L.*

Family: *Umbelliferae*

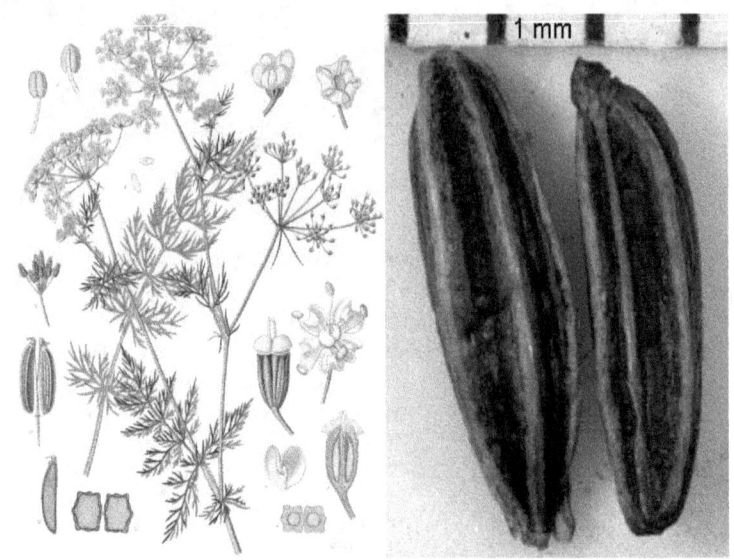

Perennial and biennial herbaceous plant

Colour: brown, or pale brown.

Odour: aromatic.

Taste: aromatic and slightly pungent.

Origin: Egypt, Morocco.

Chemical constituents:
- ✓ Volatile oil: 3-7 %: carvone, carveol and limonene.
- ✓ Fixed oils, Proteins, Sugars, Tannins and Resin.

Uses:

Lactogenic, carminative, condiment and flavoring agent.

17. Caraway fruits

Substitutes:

It is substituted with Indian dill fruits and Cuminum cyminum fruits.

Microscopical examination:

Characteristic microscopical features:

1. Fragment from the transverse cell layer(c).
2. Oil droplets (d) (with Sudan solution).

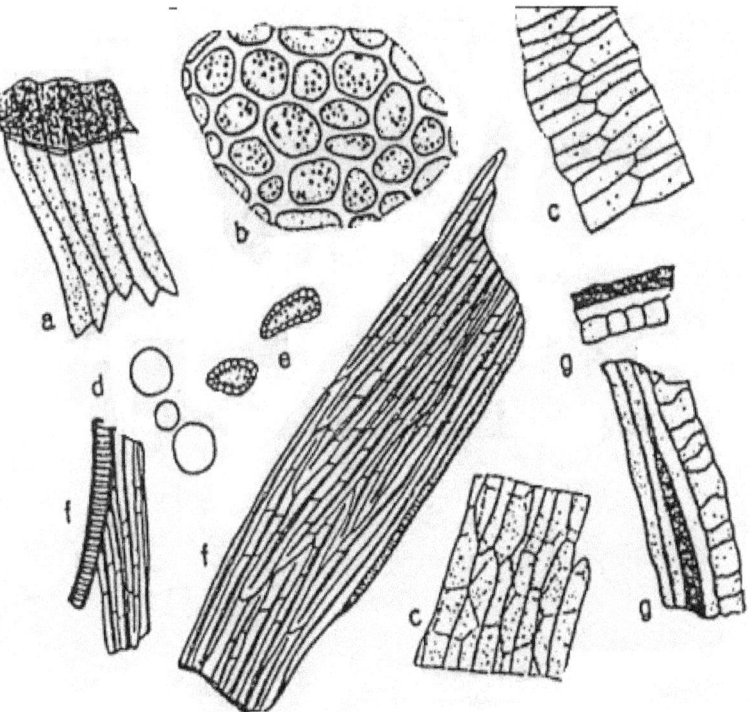

a) Fragment with the pointed end of transverse cells of the endocarp and yellow brown schizogenous secretory duct, transverse cells markedly long, not very numerous.

17. Caraway fruits

b) Fragment from the endosperm with minute calcium oxalate druses, cell walls swell strongly in chloral hydrate, very numerous.
c) Fragment from the transverse cell layer.
d) Oil droplets, numerous.
e) Isolated stone cells from the vicinity of the vascular bundles, rare
f) Sclerenchymal fiber fragment with adhering vessel from the ribs
g) Fragment from the transverse cell layer from the side with dark secretory duct.

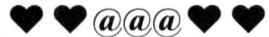

18. FENNEL FRUITS: FOENICULI FRUCTUS

Latin name: *Foeniculum vulgare L.*

Family: *Umbelliferae*

Perennial herb with yellow flowers.

Fruits colour: greenish yellow or greenish brown.

Odor: aromatic.

Taste: Aromatic and sweet.

Origin: Mediterranean region.

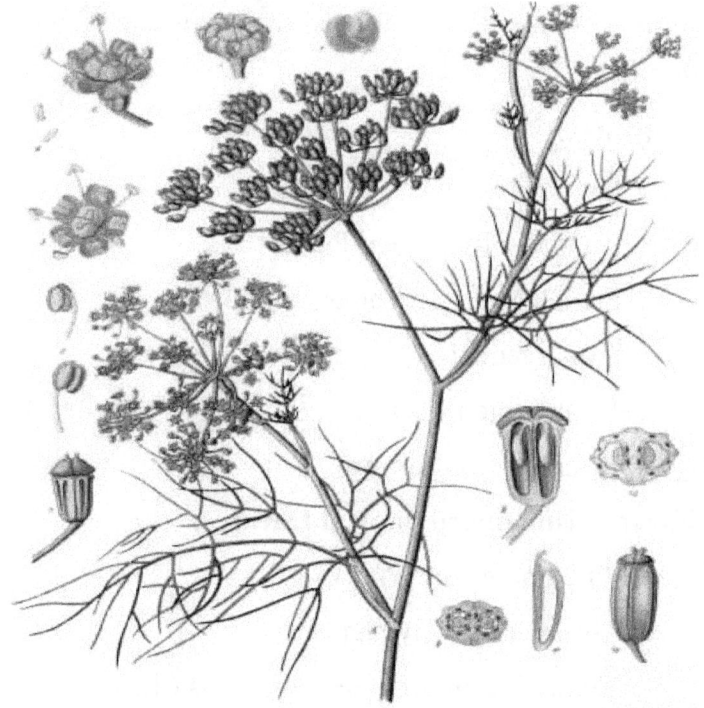

Foeniculum vulgare

18. Fennel Fruits

Chemical Constituents

Volatile oil: Fenchone, Anethole and limonene.

Uses:

1. Carminative.

2. Antispasmodic.

3. Flavoring agent.

4. Sedative for the menstrual pains.

5. Treatment of inflamed eyes.

Adulterant:

Fennel is commonly adulterated with exhausted fennel fruits.

Substitutes:

1. Saxony fennel
2. Russia or Rumanian fennel
3. French sweet or Roman fennel
4. Indian fennel
5. Japanese fennel

Microscopical examination

Characteristic microscopical features:

1. Pitted parenchyma (a).
2. Corner collenchyma (c).
3. Yellowish oil droplets, numerous (d).
4. Endosperm with minute calcium oxalate rosettes (e).

18. Fennel Fruits

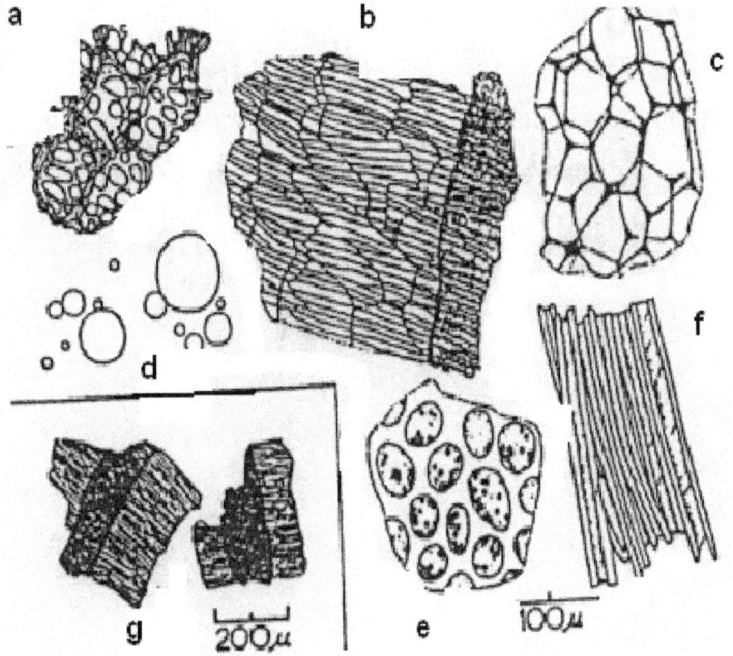

a) Pitted parenchyma (denated cells) from the mesocarp.
b) Parquet cells of the inner integument epidermis with subjacent parenchyma, on the right, residual oil duct (fragment of a schizogenous duct by epithelial cells).
c) Corner collenchyma near conducting vascular bundle with brown- red cell walls.
d) Yellowish oil droplets, numerous.
e) Endosperm fragment with minute calcium oxalate rosettes, hyaline, thick cell walls.

18. Fennel Fruits

f) Fragment of broken sclerenchymal fiber from the carophore, rare, not characteristic.

g) Fragments from the parquet cell tissue with dark yellowish secretory ducts, evident even under low magnification.

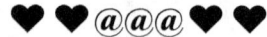

19. CARDAMOM FRUITS: FRUCTUS CARDAMOMI

Latin name: *Elettaria cardamomum White and Maeon.*

Family: *Zingiberaceae*

- Perennial small trees (2-3) m.
- The plant has very large leaves.
- Fruits form: capsule.
- Fruits color: pale green to yellow.
- Seeds: brownish black.
- Taste and odor: aromatic.
- Indigenous: India & Sri Lanka.

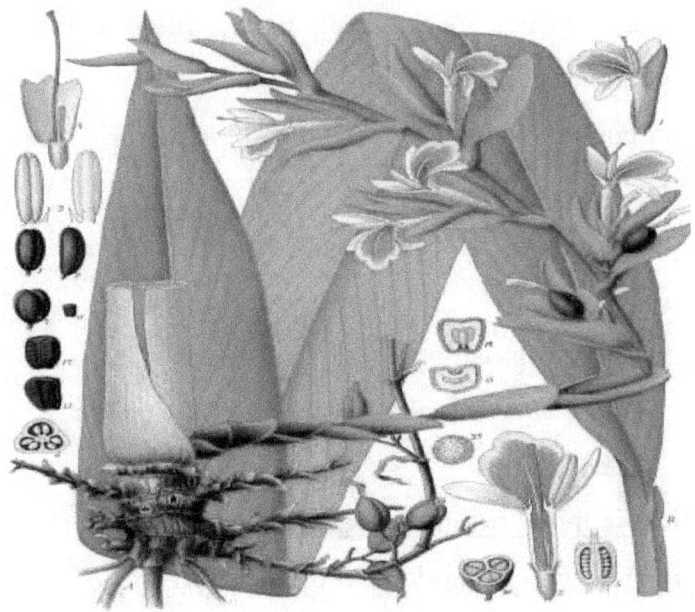

Elettaria cardamomum

19. Cardamom Fruits

Chemical constituents:

1. Volatile oil:

a. Terpenyl acetate

b. borneol

c. cineole

d. limonene

2. Fixed oil

3. Starch

Uses:

Flavoring agent, carminative, condiment, antibacterial activity and halitosis treatment.

Adulterants:

Cardamom fruits are often adulterated with orange seeds and unroasted coffee grains.

Very common adulterants of cardamom are mentioned below.

1. Long wild native cardamom (*Elettaria cardamom var. major*)
2. Korarima cardamom
3. The loose seeds of cardamom or fully ripe seeds
4. Cardamom husk

Microscopical examination

The characteristic microscopical features:

1. Stone cell layer (a1).

19. Cardamom Fruits

2. Cells from the endosperm with calcium oxalate single crystals (c).

3. Perisperm fragments containing starch (d).

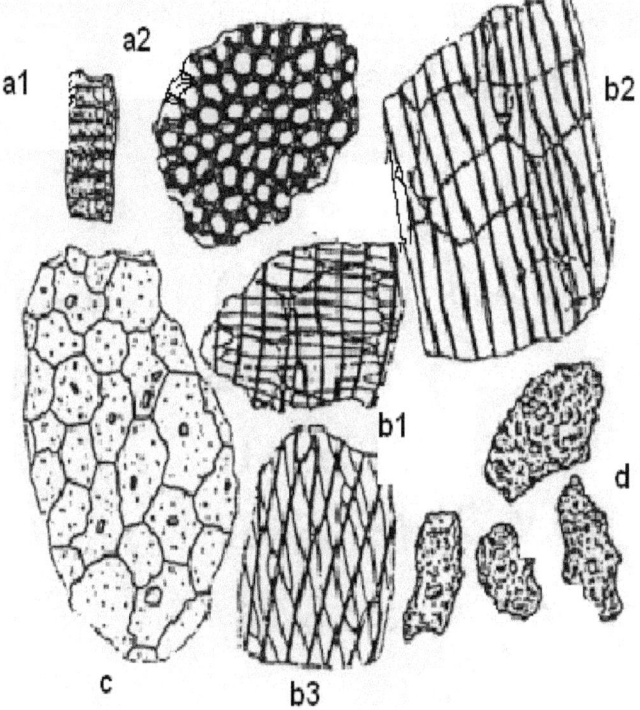

a1) Stone cell layer of the seed pod in side view, the cell walls dark

   brown.

a2) Like a1 but in top view.

b1) seed pod with lightly pitted epidermis cells, with the delicate walled cell layer, and large cells of excretory cell layer in top view.

b2) like b1 without transverse layer.

19. Cardamom Fruits

b3) like b2 without excretory cell layer.

c) Cells from the endosperm with calcium oxalate single crystals.

d) Perisperm fragments containing starch.

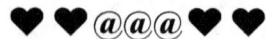

20. SAGE LEAVES: FOLIA SALVIAE

Latin name: *Salvia officinalis L.*

Family: *Labiatae*

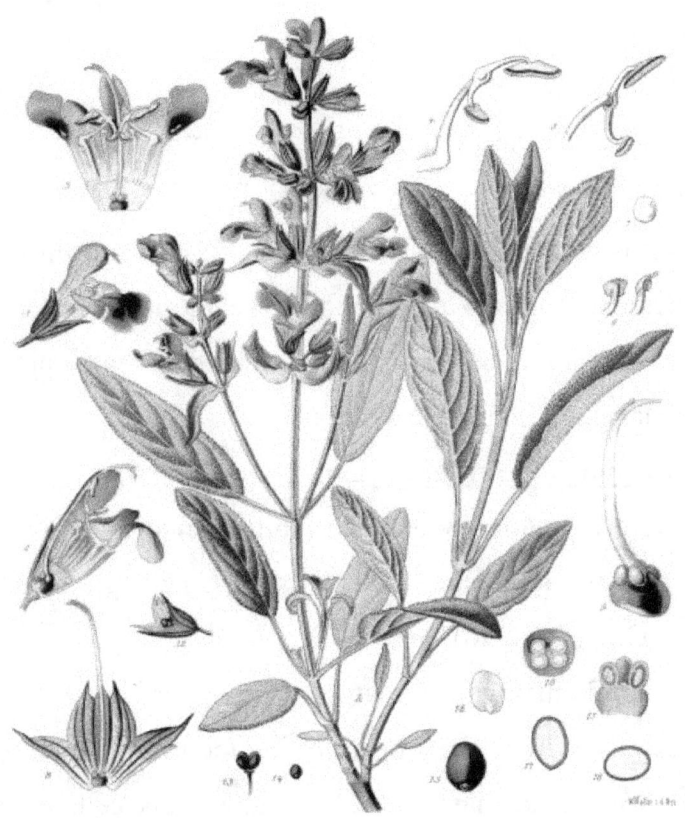

- Perennial herbaceous plant with oval leaves.
- Colour : grayish green
- Odour: aromatic /spicy.
- Taste: slightly bitter & aromatic/spicy.
- Origin : Mediterranean region

20. Sage leaves

Chemical constituents:

1- Volatile oil: a mixture of "camphor 8%, camphene 30%, cineole, thujone 50%, borneol"

2- Flavonoids

3. Ursolic acid

Uses:

Antiseptic, antispasmodic, carminative, antidandruff, flavoring agents

* Thujone acts as antioxidant, so we can use it to improve the memory (inhibits acetyl choline synthesis in the brain) and it is recommended to be used in the treatment and prophylaxes of Alzheimer's disease.

Microscopical examination:

Characteristic microscopical examinations:

1. Transparent and multicellular long hair (g).
2. Gland scale (a).
3. Epidermis with stomato and glandular hairs (b).

a) Fragment from the upper leaf epidermis in top view with glandular hair scale, stomata & stalk cells of two broken glandular hairs.

b) Fragment from the lower leaf epidermis in top view with stomata & glandular hairs.

20. Sage leaves

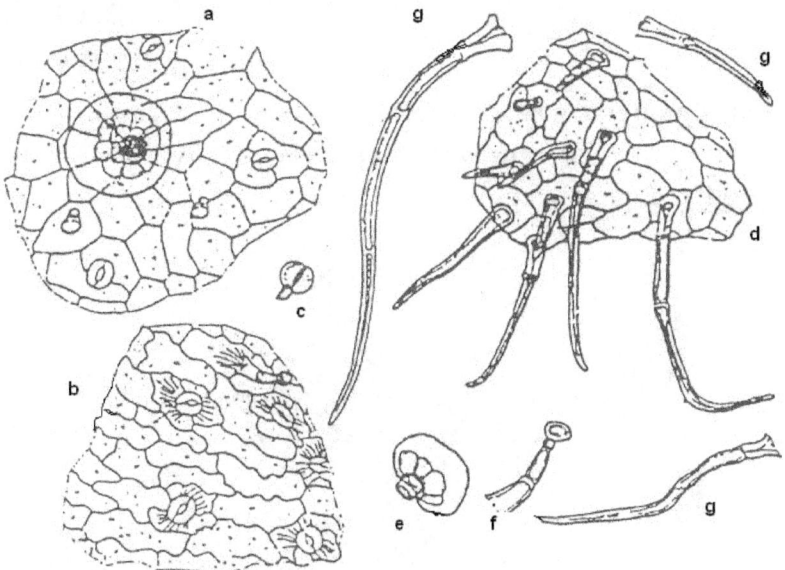

c) Glandular hair.
d) Fragment from the leaf epidermis in top view.
e) Gland scale in side view.
f) Fragment of glandular hair.
g) Multicellular hairs.

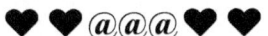

21. THYME LEAVES: FOLIA THYMI

Latin name: *Thymus vulgaris L.* (Garden Thyme)
Thymus serpylum L. (Wild Thyme)
Family: *Labiatae*

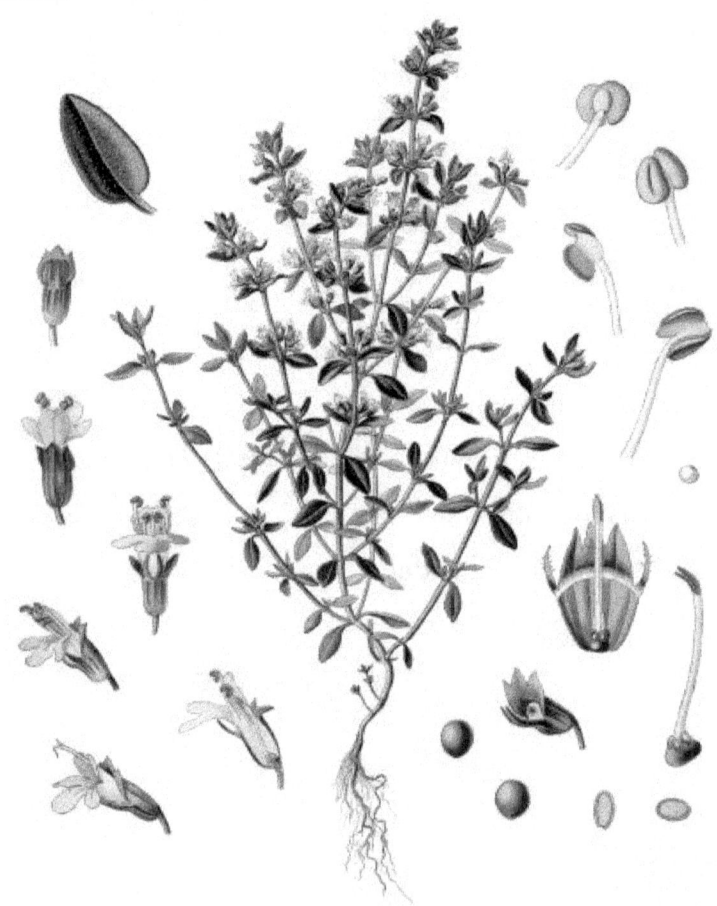

Thymus vulgaris
Garden Thyme

21. Thyme leaves:

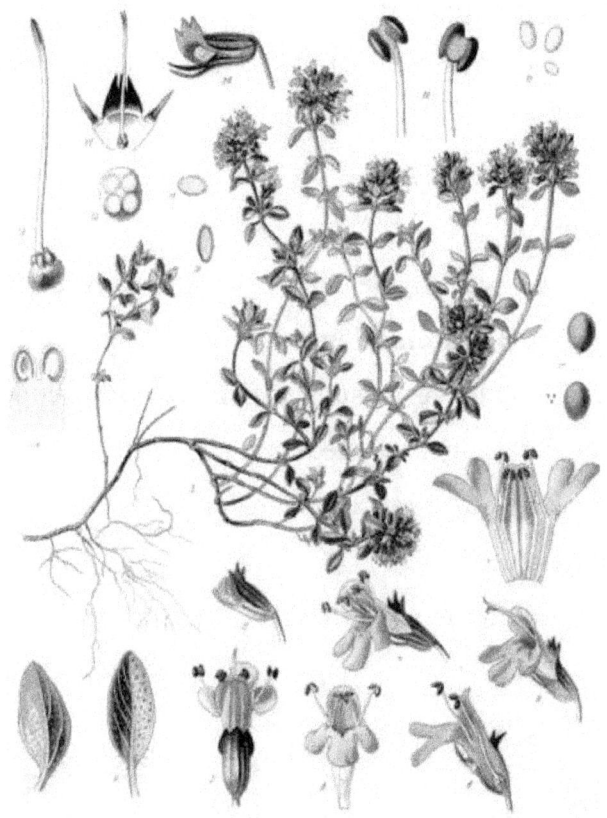

Thymus serpyllum
Wild Thyme

- Perennial herbaceous plant with oval, small and hairy leaves.
- Colour: grayish green leaves.
- Odour: aromatic.
- Taste: aromatic and slightly pungent.
- Origin: Mediterranean regions.

21. Thyme leaves:

Chemical constituents:

Volatile oils: thymol, terpenes, carvacol and carvacrol

Uses:

a) Antibacterial.

b) Anti-fungal.

c) Expectorant (as Thyme extract) (due to Carvacrol).

Microscopical examination

Characteristic leaves tissues under the microscope:

1. Multicellular thick-walled bent hairs (b).
2. Epidermis with short cortical hairs (a).
3. Gland scales (f1, f2).
4. Elongated multicellular hair (c).

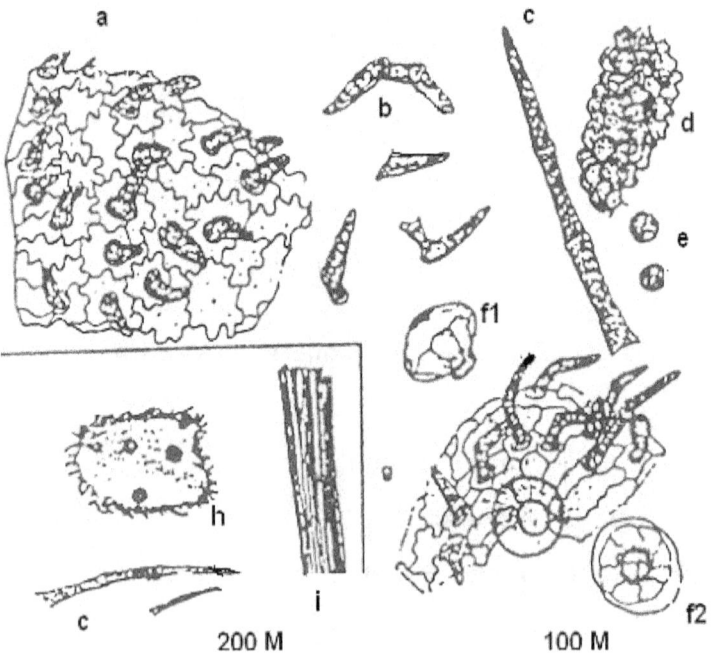

21. Thyme leaves:

a) Epidermal fragment with short conical hairs.
b) Torn, multicellular thick-walled bent hairs.
c) Fragment of an elongated multicellular hair.
d) Fragment of the papillose of a petal.
e) Pollen grains.
f 1) Gland scale in side view.
f 2) Gland scale in top view.
g) Epidermal fragment with gland scale, hairs.
h) Leaf fragment with numerous hairs and gland scales under the magnifying glass.
i) Sclerenchyma fiber bundle from the stem under the magnifying glass.

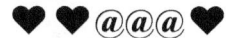

22. PEPPERMINT LEAVES: FOLIA MENTHAE

Latin name:

*Mentha piperita L. (*Garden Mint)

Mentha spicata L. (Spearmint)

Family: *Labiatae*

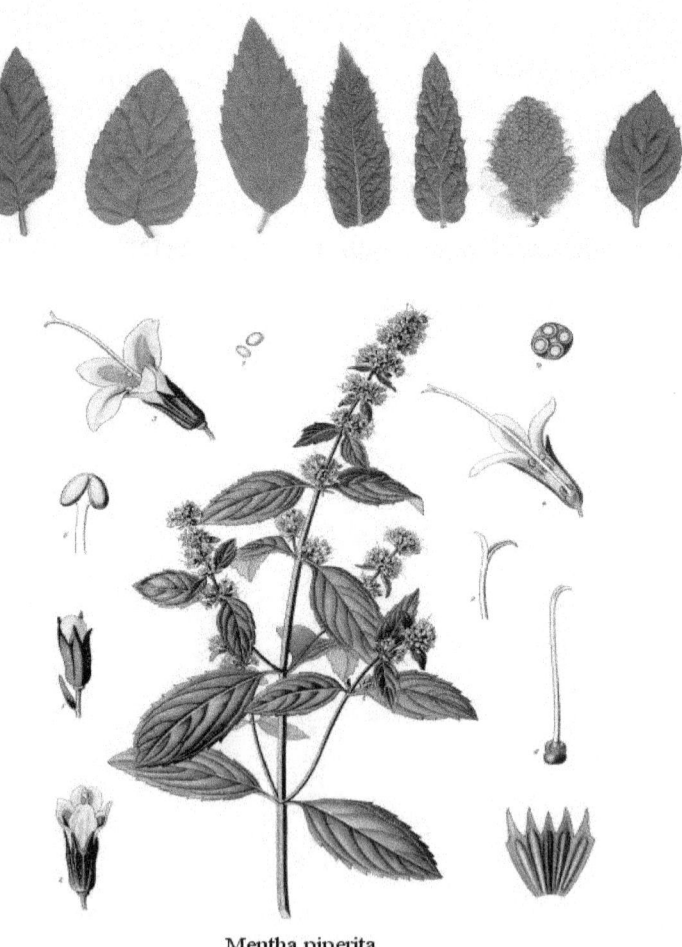

Mentha piperita

22. Peppermint Leaves

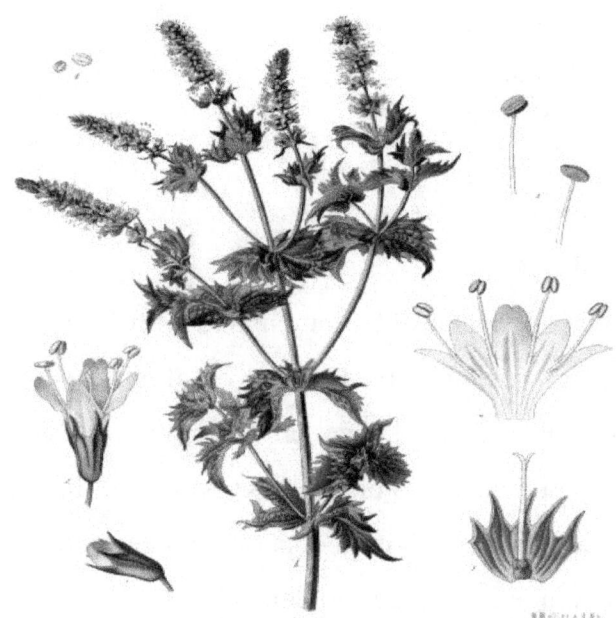

Mentha spicata

- Perennial herbaceous plant.
- It needs day time length 15-16 hours.
- The leaves are thin & dentate.
- Colour: green.
- Odor: aromatic.
- Taste: aromatic & pungent.
- Origin: Europe & Mediterranean regions.

Chemical constituents:

I. Peppermint oil (V.O) 1-2% yellow & pungent:
   1. menthol 50-90%
   2. menthone
   3. menthafurane
   4. menthyl acetate

22. Peppermint Leaves

      5. valeric acid
      6. cineole
      7. jasmone.
II.   Resins
III. Tannins

Chemical test:

Few drops of peppermint oil are mixed with 5 ml of nitric acid solution (prepared by adding 1 ml of nitric acid to 300 ml of glacial acetic acid. Heat on water bath. Within five minutes liquid develops blue colour, which on further heating deepens and shows copper colour fluorescence after sometime it becomes golden yellow.

Uses:
1. Carminative.
2. Flavoring agent (gums, tooth paste, mouth wash).
3. Internally menthol has a depressant effect on the heart.
4. Antiseptic.
5. Antipruritic.
6. Counter irritant (menthol).

Adulterant:

Mentha oil is de-mentholized and used as adulterant.

Microscopical examination

The characteristic key elements are:

22. Peppermint Leaves

1. Multicellular non-glandular hair (translucent hairs) (d).
2. Epidermis with gland scales (a).

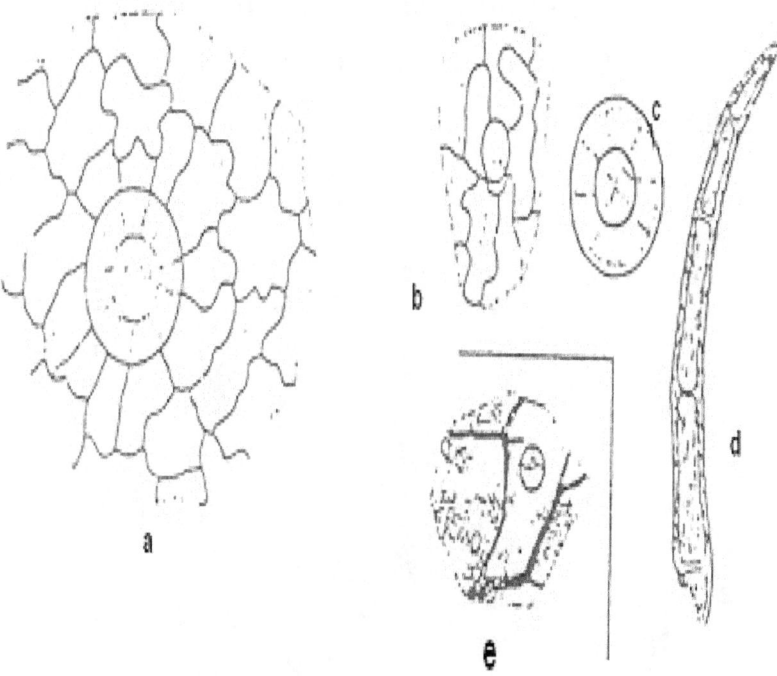

a) Epidermal fragment with gland scale.
b) Epidermal fragment with glandular hair.
c) Younger glandular hair.
d) Fragment of multicellular non-glandular hair.
e) General view.

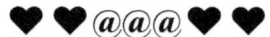

23. CAPSICUM FRUITS:
FRUCTUS CAPSICI

Latin name: *Capsicum annum*   Linn var. *longum*

Capsicum minimum   Linne

Capsicum frutescens   Linn

Family: *Solanaceae*

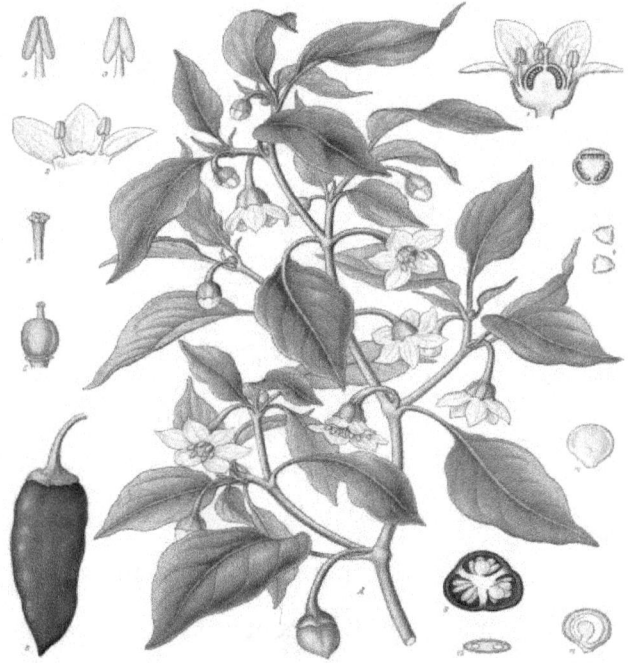

Capsicum annuum

Capsicum annum: annual herbaceous plant, fruits: 3-12 cm long fruits.

Capsicum minimum: perennial herbaceous plant, fruits: 1 – 3 cm.

23. Capsicum Fruits

Fruits

Colour: red to orange.

Odour: characteristic, irritant for mucus membrane.

Taste: pungent "strong ".

Origin: Mexico, India.

Seeds

Colour: white, yellowish white.

Chemical constituents:

1- Phenolic substance: capsaicin 0.02 % (pungent principle).

2- α & β carotene.

3- Vitamin C.

4- Fixed oil.

5- Flavonoid glycoside "capsanthin ".

Identification test:

The pungency of capsicum is not destroyed by boiling it with 2% solution of sodium hydroxide. But it is destroyed by oxidizing agents like potassium permanganate.

Uses:

Eternally: stomachic, condiment, carminative.

Externally: counter irritant, rubefacient.

Microscopical examination:

Key elements:

1. Seed shell epidermis with mesenteric cells (a).

23. Capsicum Fruits

2. The inner epidermis of the fruit with marked pitted rosulate cells (b).
3. Oil droplets, characterized by red colour (c).

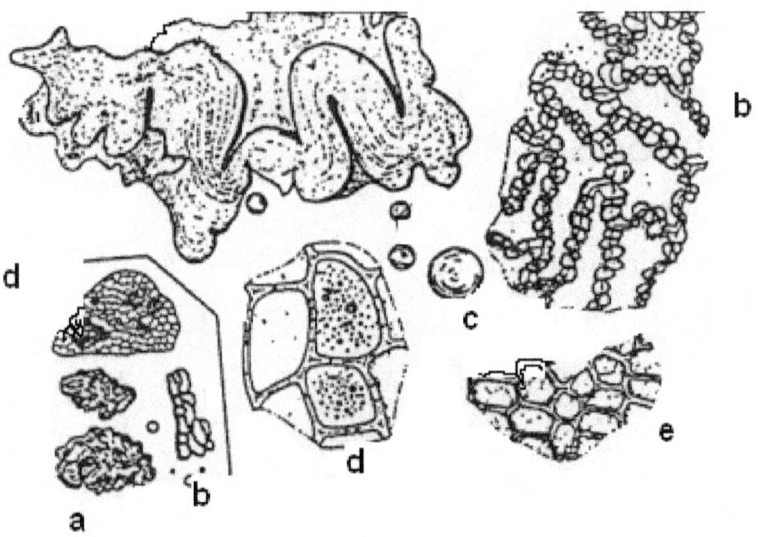

a) Fragment from the seed shell epidermis with mesenteric cells, cell wall very undulated, side wall markedly thickened & stratified, slightly greenish.
b) Fragment from the inner epidermis of the fruit with marked pitted rosulate cells, very characteristic.
c) Oil droplets, characteristic by red colour.
d) Cells from the outer epidermis in top view.
e) Fragment from the endosperm.

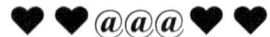

24. VASAKA:
ADHATODA, ADULSA, MALABAR NUT

Latin name: *Adhatoda vasica*

Family: Acanthaceae

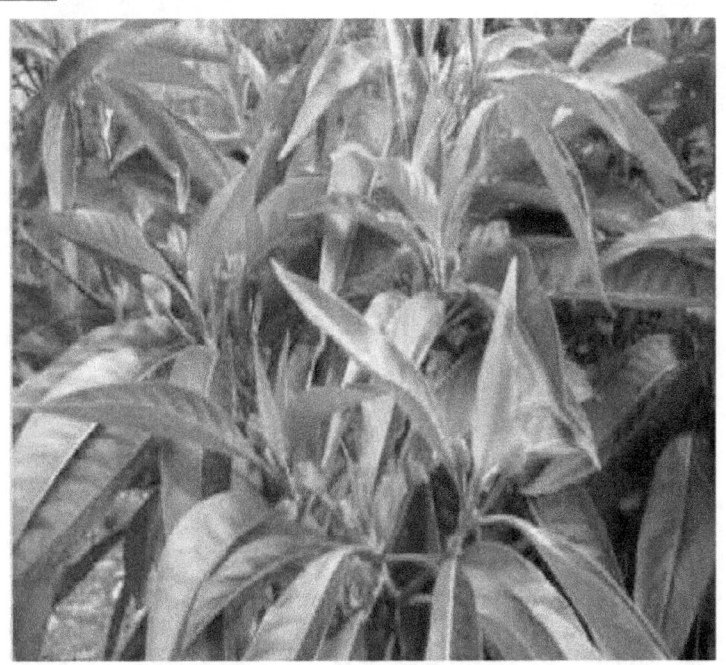

Simple, ex-stipulate, petiolate, entire, glabrous, lanceolate, acute, reticulate-unicostate.

Colour: Greenish or greyish green
Odour: characteristic
Taste: bitter

Chemical constituents:

Vasaka leaves contain quinazoline alkaloids such as vasicine, vasicinone and 6-hydroxy vasicine. Biochemically, vasicine is oxidised to its ketonic derivative

24. Vasaka:

vasicinone, which exerts the bronchodilator activity. The drug also contains volatile oil, betain and vasakin. Vasaka also contains adhatodic acid.

Uses:

- Vasaka syrup acts as an Expectorant
- Bronchodilator
- Large doses of vasaka powder causes irritation and cause vomitting and diarrhoea
- Vasicine shows oxytocic property like oxytocin and methyl ergotamine
- Vasicine also has abortificient activity due to the release of prostaglandins
- Bromhexine hydrochloride is a synthetic derivative of vasicine. This changes the structure of bronchial secretions and reduces viscosity of sputum

In T.S., the leaf shows dorsiventral structure — presence of both upper and lower epidermis of which lower epidermis contain caryophyllaceous stomata, presence of multicellular trichomes, and glandular hairs on upper epidermis, presence of palisade and spongy mesophyll cells, palisade layers containing cystolith, vascular bundles surrounded by pericycle, xylem and phloem present side by side, presence of oil globules and calcium-oxalate crystals in the mesophyll cells.

24. Vasaka:

Microscopical examination:

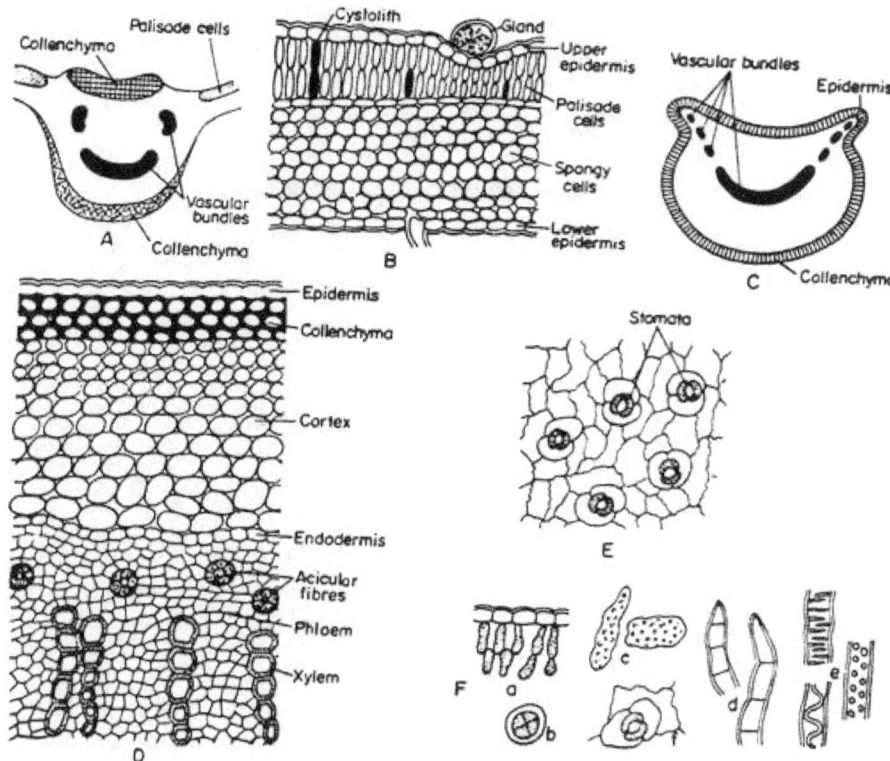

Presence of epidermal fragments with caryophyllaceous stomata, glandular and multicellular hairs, cystolith in palisade layers, oil-containing parenchymatous cells.

A-B) T.S of leaf

C-D) T.S. of petiole

E) surface view of lower epidermis showing stomata

F) Elements from powder of leaf

a) Upper epidermis and palisade in T.S.

b) Glandular trichome

24. Vasaka:

c) Cystolith

d) covering trichomes

e) vessels

f) Caryophyllaceous stomata

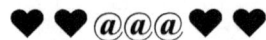

25. RAUWOLFIA: SARPAGANDHA, SERPENTINA ROOT, CHHOTACHAND

Latin name: *Rauwolfia serpentina*

Family: Apocynaceae

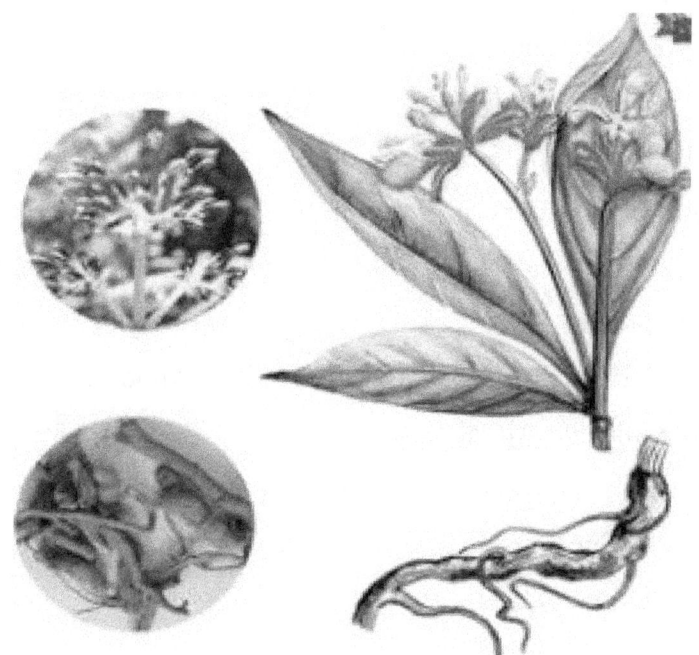

(i) External features of roots and rhizomes are nearly similar but rhizomes can be made out by the presence of small central pith.

(ii) Drug consists of mostly small pieces, which are 2 to 15 cm long and 3 to 22 mm diameter.

(iii) Pieces are cylindrical, slightly tapering and tortuous.

(iv) Outer surface is greyish yellow, pale brown or brown.

25. Rauwolfia

(v) Fracture short.

(vi) Fracture surface show yellowish to brown bark and dense pale yellow radiating wood with 2 to 8 annular rings occupying nearly three fourth of the diameter.

(vii) Odour: Odourless

(viii) Taste: bitter.

Chemical constituents:

i. Alkaloids- Indole alkaloids (1.5 or 3%) present.

ii. Weakly basic Indole type (pH 7 to 7.5)

iii. Reserpine group – Reserpine, Rescinnamine, deserpidine.

iv. Tertiary indoline alkaloids (pH-8). Ajmaline group- Ajmaline and Ajmalicine.

v. Strongly basic anhydronium bases (pH-11).

vi. Serpentine group – Serpentine, Serpentinine and Alsotonine.

Chemical tests:

1. A red coloration along the medullary rays is observed when the freshly fractured surface is treated with concentrated nitric acid.

2. Reserpine shows violet red colour when treated with solution of vanillin in acetic acid.

25. Rauwolfia

Uses:

1. Rauwolfia is used as hypotensive and tranquillizer.
2. Reserpine being the main alkaloid is responsible for the activity and is used in anxiety condition and other neuropsychoiatric diseases.
3. Sedative – calm down activities and excitement (reserpine group).
4. Stimulates the central of peripheral nervous systems (Ajmaline group).
5. The decoction of root is used to increase uterine contraction in difficult cases.
6. The extract is used for intestinal disorders and as anthelmintic bitter tonic and febrifuge.

Substitutes and adulterants:

The following species of rauwolfia are substituted for genuine drug.

R. vomitoria

R. canescens

R micrantha

Adulterants:

R. densitiflora and *R. perakensis*

25. Rauwolfia

Microscopical characters (T.S.):

T. S. of the root presents a circular outline with typical stratified cork and other secondary features. Following are the tissues seen from the periphery to the center.

1. Periderm:

a. Cork (Phellum):

Stratified, consists of alternating bands- of smaller, suberized and un-lignified cell up to 8 to 10 raw in radial depth- larger, suberized but lignified cell upto 5 to 7 raw in radial depth.

b. Phellogen:

Indistinct but is seen as a narrow layer of thin walled cells,

c. Phelloderm:

5 to 7 layers, immediately below the phloem, cell is arranged in the radial rows whereas away from phloem, cell is oval and has intercullar spaces. Phelloderm contains abundant starch grains (with triradiate hilum) and typical twin prisms of calcium oxalate.

2. Secondary phloem:

Is transverse by conspicuous medullary rays. Phloem consists of sieve tubes, companion cells and phloem parenchyma. Starch grains and calcium oxalate prism occurs throughout the phloem tissue.

25. Rauwolfia

3. Secondary xylem:

It is also transverse by well develop medullary rays. Xylem consists of vessels, wood fibres and lignified parenchyma. The vessels appear rounded, polygonal or at times radially elongated and occurs inner single or in pairs. Xylem fibres appear as rounded and polygonal structure with thick lignified walls. Typical oxalate prism and starch grains resembling those of the phelloderm and phloem occur freely in the wood parenchyma.

4. Medullary rays:

It runs radially from the center to the cortex through the phloem. Rays in the xylem region are lignified, pitted and are 1 to 5 cells wide although uniseriate rays are prominent. In the phloem region the ray cells are not lignified. Starch and typical oxalate prisms are in the medullary ray cells.

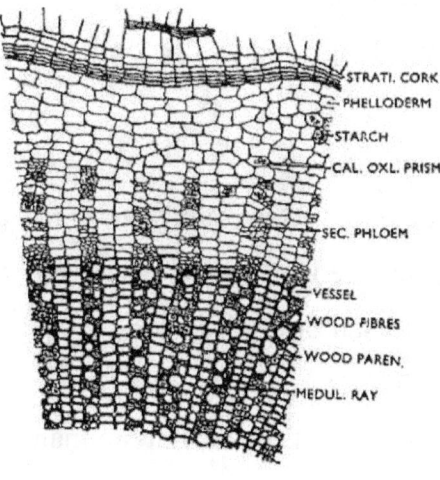

25. Rauwolfia

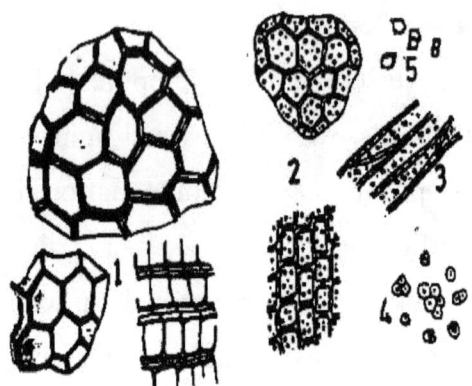

Powder analysis of Rauwolfia:

1. Cork:

Stratified cork in several layers appearing like benzene rings

2. Parenchyma:

Pitted and lignified parenchymatous cells of the xylem parenchyma and medullary ray cells.

3. Wood elements:

Vessels few, long and with oblique end walls and perforations.

4. Starch granules:

Largely simple but compound ones are also known to occur. Granules are fairly large, possessing a distinct hilum in the form of a star or a split.

5. Calcium oxalate:

Crystals in the form of prisms but not many in number.

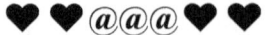

26. DATURA: ANGEL'S TRUMPET

Latin name: *Datura metel*

Family: Solanaceae

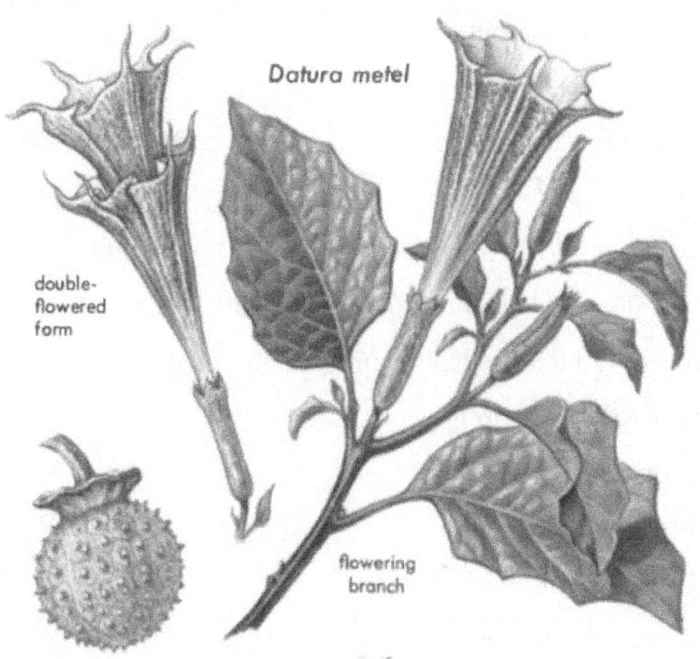

Leaves:

(i) Sub glabrous spreading herb with cylindrical stem.

(ii) Shape single triangular ovate.

(iii) Base unequal

(iv) Margin toothed.

Flower:

(i) Solitary, funnel shaped large and tubular, 7.5 to 9 cm length.

26. Datura

(ii) Corolla 15 to 18 cm length, 10-12.5 cm across at the mouth

Fruit:

Sub-globose capsule covered with short and blunt spines, 2.5 to 3.2 cm diameter nodding or sub erect.

D. Metel Var. Fastuosa:

While many characters of this plant are similar to those of D. Metel the stem, branches, main veins of leaves and also flowers are violet or purple coloured. Double- flowered and triple flowered forms (outer corolla 5 teeth and inner corolla 6-10 teeth) also occur, though not so common.

Chemical constituents:

1. Tropane alkaloids
    a. Hyoscyamine
    b. Scopolamine (hyoscine)
2. Fastudine and fastunine,
3. Fastusic acid, alantoin.
4. Ascorbic acid, etc.

Chemical Tests:

1. **Vitali- Morin reactions:**

    The drug is treated concentrated nitric acid, filtered and solution is evaporated to dryness. To the residue, add acetone and methanolic potassium hydroxide solution, violet colour is produced due to Tropane derivative.

26. Datura

2. On addition of silver nitrate solution to solution of hyoscine hydrobromide, yellowish white precipitate is formed, which is insoluble in nitric acid, but soluble in dilute ammonia.

Uses:

1. Mydriatic (dilation of the pupil).
2. Antispasmodic (a drug that counteracts a sudden, violent, involuntary muscular contraction)
3. Antimuscarinic effect (acts peripherally to produce parasympathetic inhibition).
4. Antisialagogue (a drug that arrest the flow of excess of saliva)
5. Cerebral sedative (reduce excitement)

Microscopical characters:

Lamina:

Upper epidermis:

They are single layered, cells rectangular with cuticularized outer walls. Trichomes, both covering and glandular are seen. Covering trichomes are uniseriate, multicellular, warty and blunt at the apex. Glandular trichomes are made up to a stalk of one cell and a 2 to 4 celled glandular head.

26. Datura

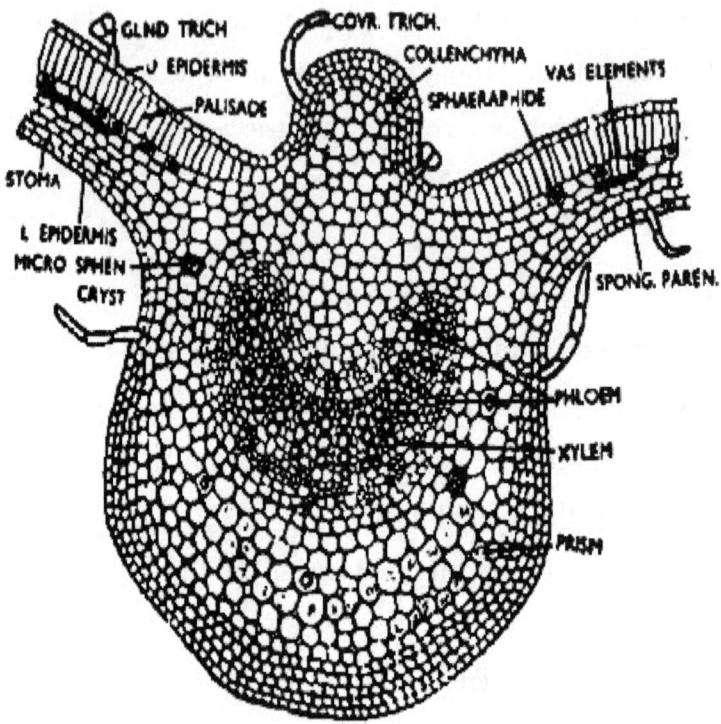

Mesophyll:

It is differentiated into palisade and spongy parenchyma.

Palisade:

It is a single layered, compact and cells radially elongated.

Spongy parenchyma:

They are many layered, loosely arranged with intercellular spaces. Sphaeraphides, microsphenoidal crystals and vascular strands are found in the upper layers of spongy parenchyma.

26. Datura

Lower epidermis:

It is identical to upper epidermis. Stomata and numerous trichomes are seen on the lower epidermis.

Midrib:

The epidermis layers of lamina are continuous in the midrib region also. Strips of collenchymas appear below the upper and above the lower epidermis. This is followed by cortical parenchyma containing prisms of calcium oxalate and microsphenoidal crystals. Embedded in the central region of the cortical parenchyma is a bicollateral bundle.

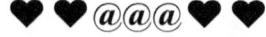

27. CARBOHYDRATES
1. Starch

Definition:

Carbohydrates: natural plant products – organic compounds consist of C, H and O.

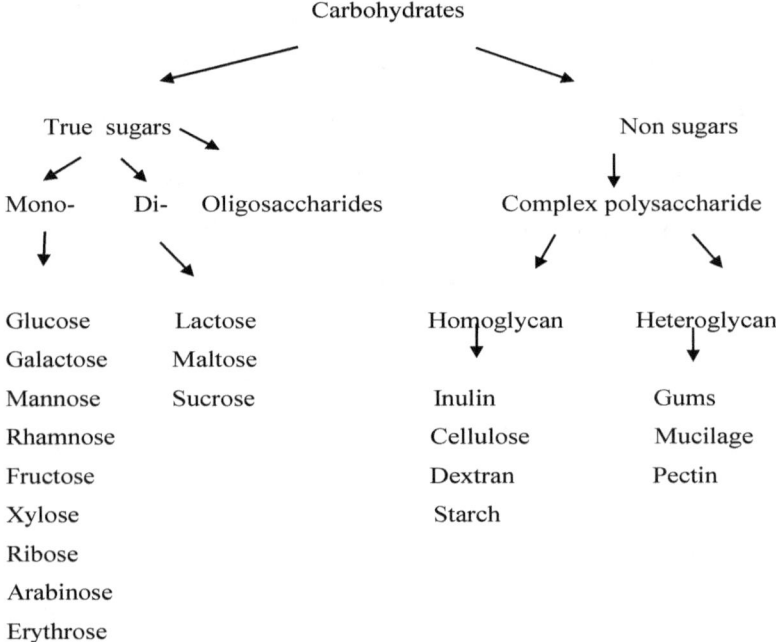

Complex polysaccharides: substances with very high molecular weight and consist of a large number of monosaccharide units linked together through glycosidic linkage.

Starch (Amylum):

Natural plant product which is a mixture of amylose (25%) and amylopectin (75%).

27. Carbohydrates

Amylose:
- Linear molecule consists of 250 – 300 units of α – D – glucose units linked together through α – 1,4 glycosidic linkage.
- More water soluble than amylopectin
- Amylose + I_2 → blue color

Amylopectin:
- Branched molecule consists of more than 1000 units of α- D – glucose linked together through α – 1,4 and α- 1,6 glycosidic linkage.
- Amylopectin is less water soluble than amylose.
- Amylopectin + I_2 → violet color

Plants containing starch:
- ✓ Cereal seeds contain 50- 65 % starch
- ✓ Ginger rhizomes 50% starch.
- ✓ Potato tubers 80- 90% starch.

Commercial sources of starch:

1. Corn starch: isolated from the caryopses of ***Zea mays L.*** – (***Graminae***)

2. Wheat starch: isolated from the caryopses of ***Triticum aestivum L.*** – (***Graminae***)

3. Rice starch: isolated from the caryopses of ***Oryza sativa L.*** – (***Graminae***)

27. Carbohydrates

4. Potato starch: isolated from the tubers of *Solanum tuberosum L.* – (*Solanaceae*)

Properties of Starch:

1. White mass powder, odorless with starchy taste
2. Insoluble in water and form colloidal solution with water.
3. Starch + I_2 → Deep blue color.
4. Starch + NaOH or chloral hydrate → gelatinization
5. Starch + H_2O → gel (with heat)
6. Corn starch and wheat starch have neutral pH

Rice starch has slightly alkaline pH.

Potato starch has slightly acidic pH.

Identification tests for starch:

1) Give positive reaction with Fehling's solution test:
   Starch + HCl (hydrolysis) + NaOH (neutralization) + Fehling's solution → Red colour
2) Give positive reaction with Molisch's test
   Starch + H_2SO_4 + α- naphthol → Purple ring
3) Starch + H_2O → gel (jelly form) with heat
4) Starch + I_2→ deep blue → colour disappears (with heating) → the colour reappears with cooling.

The general uses:

1. Nutritive.
2. Demulcent.

27. Carbohydrates

3. Pharmaceutical uses as tablets filler and binder.
4. Antipruritic: Baby paste®-(Vitamed company) used in case of diaper rash, skin irritation (ZnO, Starch).
5. Industrial uses: papers, clothes.
6. Antidote in case of poisoning from Iodine.

Microscopical characters:

I. Potato starch
- Central and eccentric hilum (dot shape)
- The horse shoe-shaped hila are eccentrically situated, small and unapparent
- Clear striations(rings are clearly evident)
- Mussel- shaped

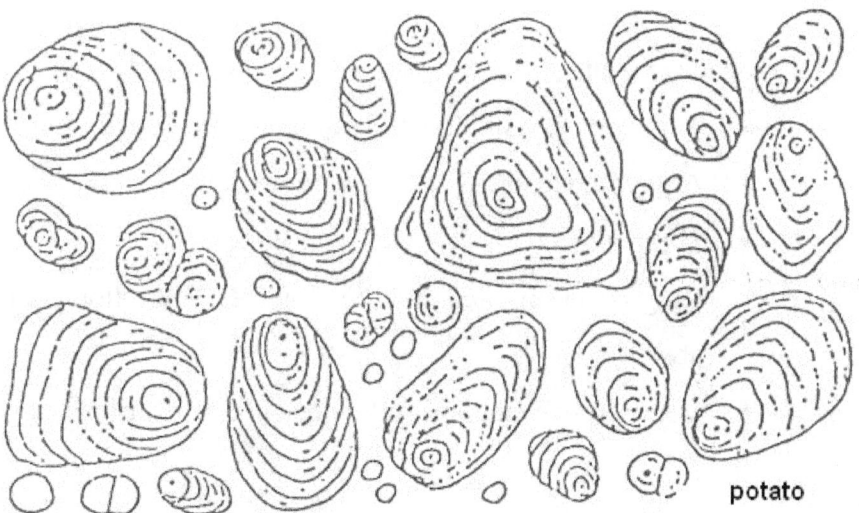
potato

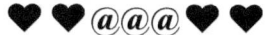

27. Carbohydrates

2. RICE PLANT

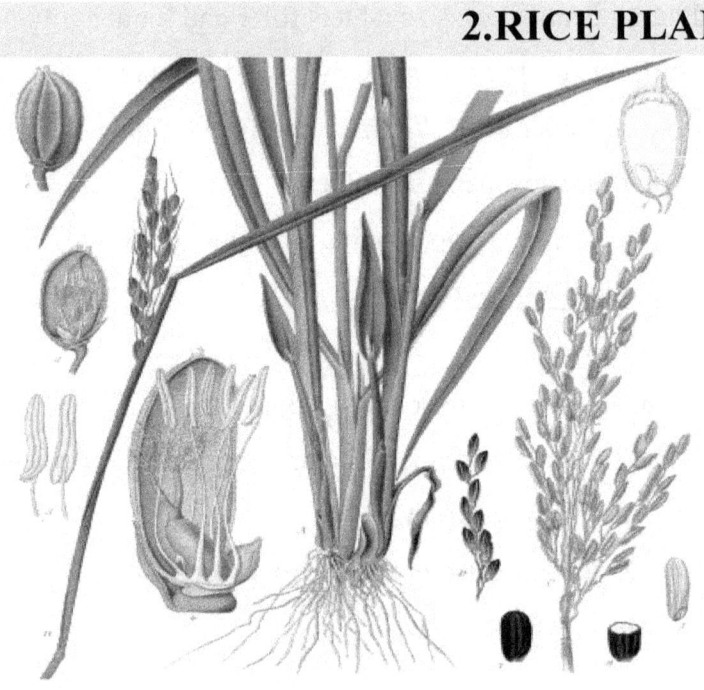

II. Rice starch

- They are very small, polyhedral and polygonal grains
- Aggregated from 2 – 150 component
- Sharp angles
- Rings and hila cannot be detected (Striations are absent)
- Very rare we can detect the presence of centric hila.

27. Carbohydrates

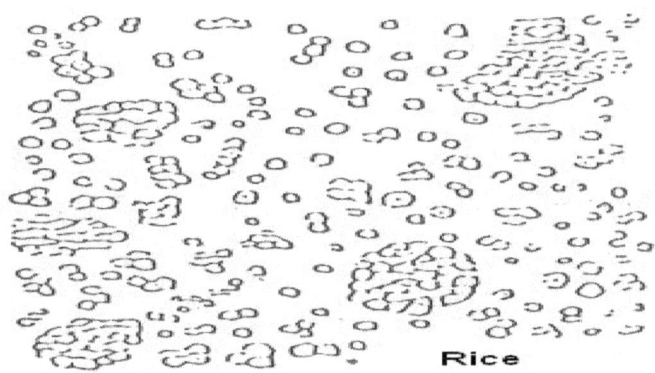

Wheat plant

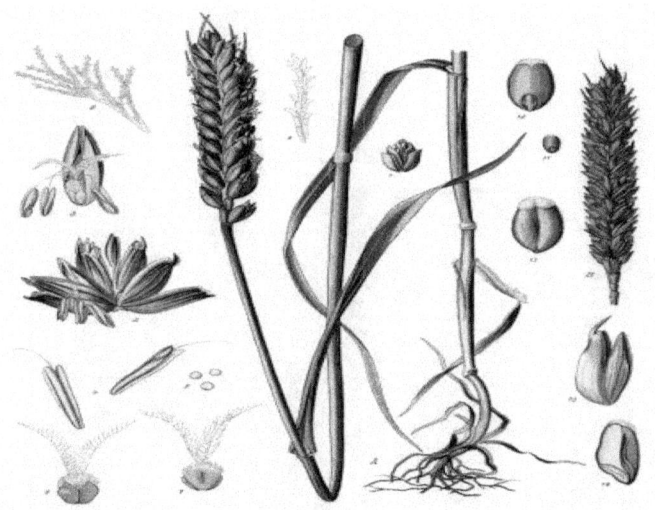

III. Wheat starch

- Contain large granules.
- Lenticular.
- Smaller ones globular.
- Hilum is centric.

27. Carbohydrates

- Faint striations.
- Transition sizes are rare.

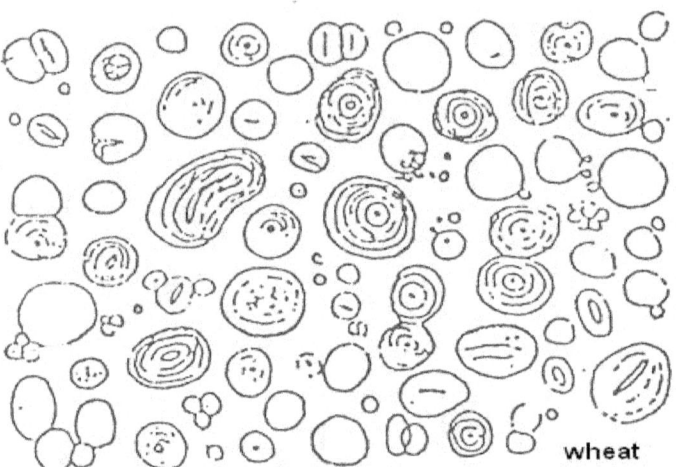
wheat

Corn plant

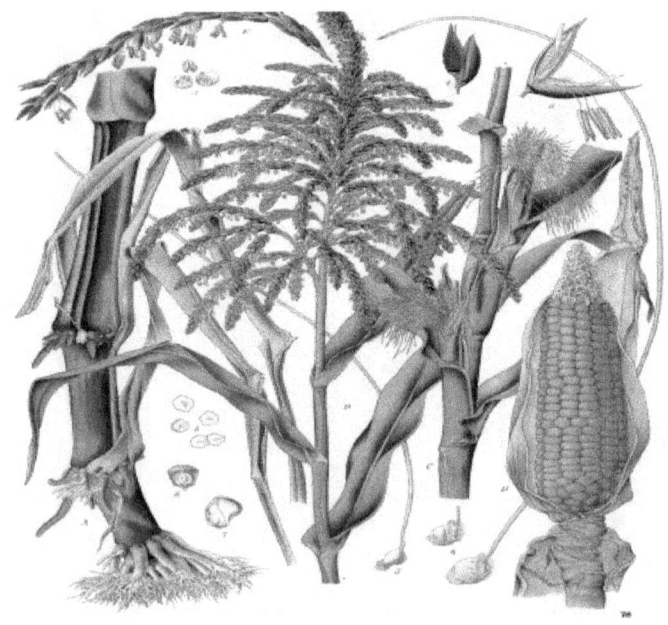

27. Carbohydrates

IV. Corn starch

- Rings (striations) are usually absent.
- Spheroidal and polygonal.
- Polyhydral
- The usually stellate hila can often be found
- X-Y hilum

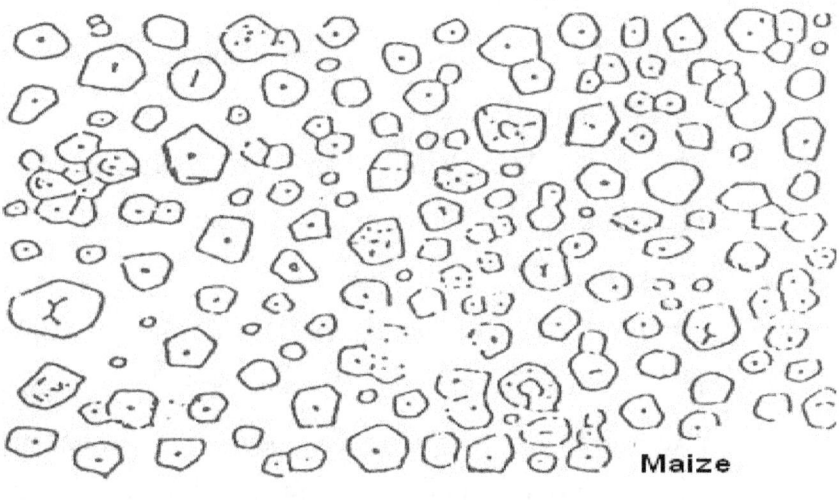
Maize

♥ ♥ @@@ ♥ ♥

BIBLIOGRAPHY

1) Evans WC. Trease and Evans Pharmacognosy, 15th edition, Harcourt Publisher limited, London, 2002.
2) James E, Robbers, Marilyn K, Speedie, Varro E. Tyler Pharmacognosy and Pharmacobiotechnology, Pennsylvania, USA, 1996.
3) Wallis TE. Text book of Pharmacognosy, 5th edition, Shahdara, Delhi, India, 1985
4) Mohamed Ali, Jamia hamdard, Text book of Pharmacognosy, 2nd edition, Hamdard Nagar, New delhi, India, 1998.
5) Makboul A, Makboul, Afaf M, Abdel Baky. Pharmacognosy, Amman – Jordan, 1998.
6) Jean Bruneton. Pharmacognosy, Phytochemistry, Medicinal Plants, Lavoisier Publisher, England, 1995.
7) Kokate CK, Purohit AP, Gokhale SB. Pharmacognosy, 43rd edition, Nirali Prakashan, Pune, India, 2009.

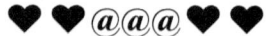

Notes

www.ingramcontent.com/pod-product-compliance
Lightning Source LLC
Chambersburg PA
CBHW070302230526
45470CB00002B/692